# THE SCIENCE OF THE
# TOUR DE FRANCE

# THE SCIENCE OF THE
# TOUR DE FRANCE

## Training secrets of the world's best cyclists

## JAMES WITTS

# BLOOMSBURY
LONDON · OXFORD · NEW YORK · NEW DELHI · SYDNEY

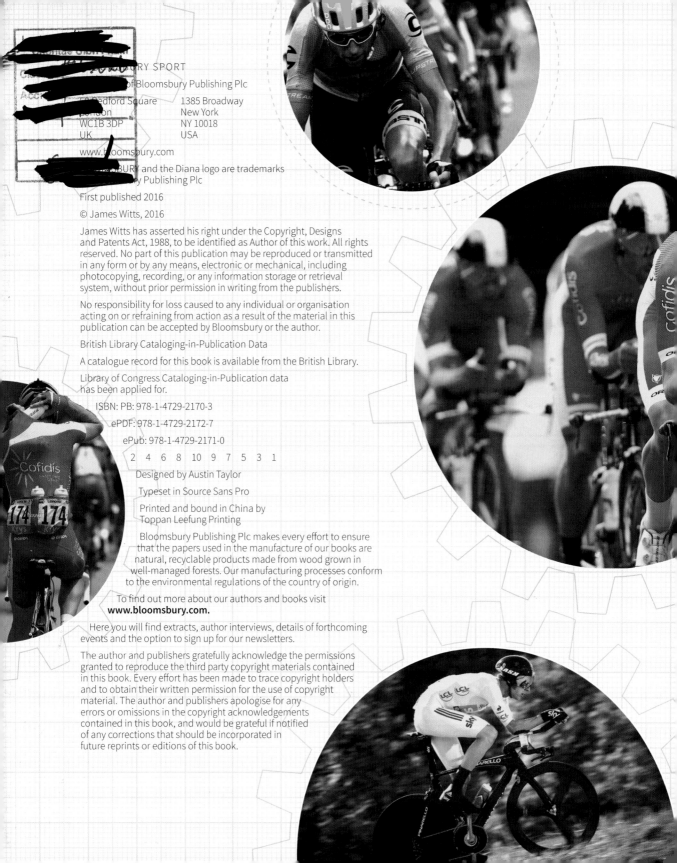

BLOOMSBURY SPORT
An imprint of Bloomsbury Publishing Plc

50 Bedford Square          1385 Broadway
London                     New York
WC1B 3DP                   NY 10018
UK                         USA

www.bloomsbury.com

BLOOMSBURY and the Diana logo are trademarks
of Bloomsbury Publishing Plc

First published 2016

British Library Cataloging-in-Publication Data

A catalogue record for this book is available from the British Library.

Library of Congress Cataloging-in-Publication data
has been applied for.

ISBN: PB: 978-1-4729-2170-3

ePDF: 978-1-4729-2172-7

ePub: 978-1-4729-2171-0

2  4  6  8  10  9  7  5  3  1

Designed by Austin Taylor

Typeset in Source Sans Pro

Printed and bound in China by
Toppan Leefung Printing

Bloomsbury Publishing Plc makes every effort to ensure
that the papers used in the manufacture of our books are
natural, recyclable products made from wood grown in
well-managed forests. Our manufacturing processes conform
to the environmental regulations of the country of origin.

To find out more about our authors and books visit
**www.bloomsbury.com.**

Here you will find extracts, author interviews, details of forthcoming
events and the option to sign up for our newsletters.

The author and publishers gratefully acknowledge the permissions
granted to reproduce the third party copyright materials contained
in this book. Every effort has been made to trace copyright holders
and to obtain their written permission for the use of copyright
material. The author and publishers apologise for any
errors or omissions in the copyright acknowledgements
contained in this book, and would be grateful if notified
of any corrections that should be incorporated in
future reprints or editions of this book.

# CONTENTS

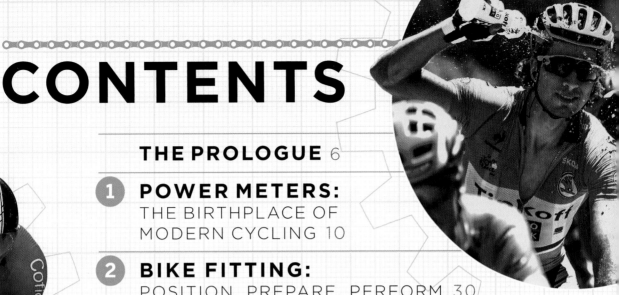
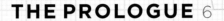
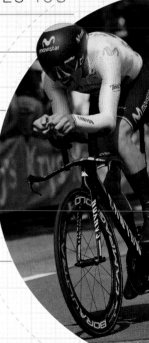

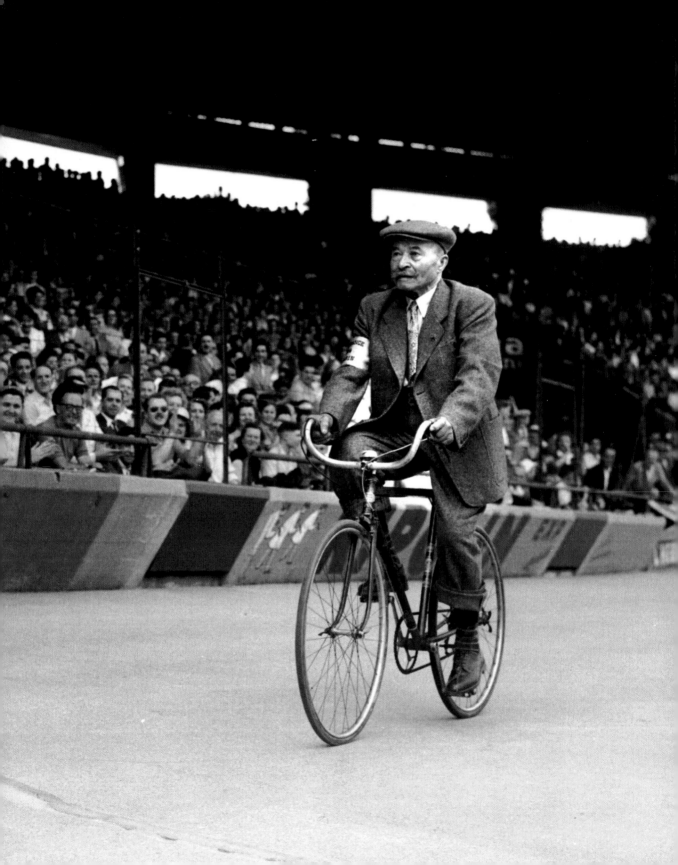

# THE PROLOGUE

**Maurice Garin won his first professional race** in 1893. The 22-year-old Frenchman had worked as a chimney sweep seven years earlier before opening a bike shop with his brothers François and César. But he loved to race. So he worked. And raced. That first victory came in a 24-hour race in Paris and highlighted the impact a good bike has on performance – Garin had sold his first bike before the race and replaced it with a much lighter model. It still weighed more than 16kg, but after riding 701km in 24 hours, he crossed the line 49 minutes ahead of his nearest rival.

Garin not only had the distance to contend with – there was the cold, too. The race took place in February, which explains the Frenchman's race nutrition plan that included eight cooked eggs, 45 lamb cutlets, an uncertain number of oysters, and all washed down with 7 litres of tea and 19 litres of hot chocolate.

Ten years of racing later, Garin's equipment and nutrition choice was equally as rudimentary, but that didn't stop him winning the inaugural Tour de France in 1903. He ticked off the six-stage race – stage distances ranging from 268km to 471km – in 94 hours, 33 minutes and 14 seconds, beating countryman Lucien Pothier by nearly three hours. He did so with a minimal support staff – Garin's friend Delattre 'preparing sustenance', though he did have a soigneur to ease aching muscles.

In 2015, Chris Froome won his second Tour de France aboard his carbon-fibre Pinarello Dogma F8, which hit the scales at 6.8kg – nearly 10kg lighter. While Garin raced alone, Froome received valuable support from his eight Team Sky teammates, sending him to Paris at the end of the 21st stage in 84 hours, 46 minutes and 14 seconds, just one minute and 12 seconds clear of runner-up Nairo Quintana.

As well as the riders, Team Sky sent a support team so large that other teams complained that their fleet of vehicles was hogging the hotel car parks. Within the equipment truck, kitchen truck and support cars sat a group of men and women who provided nutritional data and mechanical and sports-science support, all in the name of peak performance.

◁ Maurice Garin, winner of the first Tour de France in 1903, taking a lap of honour in the Parc des Princes, Paris, at the finish of the 50th Tour de France, on 26th July 1953

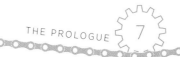

Team Sky might be the standard-bearers for science in professional cycling but other teams have cottoned on. In the past, a team's budget would have almost entirely focused on a rider's salary. In 2016, though riders' bank accounts still account for a high proportion of a team's annual budget – Tinkoff Sport's Peter Sagan and Alberto Contador are both reportedly on a salary of €4 million – teams are waking up to the fact that it's worth spending €1.9 million on a rider and €100,000 on a world-class sports scientist rather than spending €2 million purely on the rider.

Where once riders' training schedules consisted of riding until the sun disappeared, now they're based on training zones, power meters and analytical computer software. Garin's oysters have been replaced with gels that have been researched, designed and tested in laboratories.

And that's where *The Science of the Tour de France* comes in. I've spoken to the world's greatest riders about their application of science, but to really get under the skin of why they'd choose a certain depth of wheel over another or an electrolyte drink over water, I've interviewed and spent race time with the men and women in metaphorical white coats too.

Over the next 12 chapters, sports scientists, coaches and nutritionists from Tinkoff Sport, Team Sky, Movistar, Giant-Alpecin, BMC Racing and many other teams are placed under the spotlight to answer such questions as: What is the ideal altitude for a training camp? How do riders keep cool when the mercury tips over 40°C? And why on earth do Giant-Alpecin insist on drinking Slush Puppies before a time trial?

What's most exciting to me is that this is applied science. Cyclists and their support teams are testing out cutting-edge theories – and often the research is brand new. As Dr Jonathan Baker, sports scientist at Team Dimension Data told me, 'There are lots of scientists working around the world on research projects focused on subjects like "what causes fatigue?" or "how to boost power?" We tend to see an awful lot of research papers – around 10,000 are published globally every year. Your job is to pick through them and find the applicable bits, sometimes modifying the detail to extract the best bits from the research. Something might improve a physiological parameter in the lab but simply doesn't work in the world of professional cycling, which is far less controlled.'

The Tour de France is used as the hook in this book, but clearly many of the ideas and practices are applied at professional races all around the world. But with up to 90 per cent of a team's annual media coverage coming at the Tour, it's the key race for every single team. 'That's why the Tour de France is where everyone rolls out their best protocols, their best materials, best staff, best riders,' says Tinkoff Sport's former head of sports science Daniel Healey. 'The Tour is like Formula One and all that goes into aspects like choosing the right tyres to rapid pit stops. That's why nutrition, training science, gear selection – they're all on my cycling coaching menu.'

You might ask why now? Back in the late nineties and 2000s, riders raced on carbon bikes and used energy drinks but that was about it, the application of sports

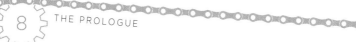

science stalling due to the greater focus on illegal performance-enhancers like EPO and blood transfusions. Why spend money on coaches, team chefs and cycle fitters when those budgets could be spent on doping and masking agents? That car boot full of narcotics in the 1998 Festina affair and Lance Armstrong's pharmaceutical cabinet didn't come cheap. It might have improved power and endurance but it all came at a (moral and human) cost.

The introduction of the blood passport – which I discuss in the altitude section – and power outputs that have dropped from the days of proven dopers like Bjarne Riis and Jan Ullrich suggests cycling is cleaner than in its recent past. Of course inevitably someone will seek a nefarious route to more speed in future, if not already, with experts suggesting that micro-dosing of EPO is now the major hurdle to a clean sport. That's why the UCI and WADA (World Anti-Doping Agency) need to invest more in the work of professors like Yannis Pitsiladis, who's designed a genetic test that could potentially detect markers of micro-dosing in an athlete's DNA. (It's not just the teams who are applying cutting-edge science, the governing bodies are onto it too.) Still, things are looking up and it could be argued that professional cycling is more open than it ever has been with groups like the Mouvement pour un Cyclisme Crédible and teams like Sky banning ex-dopers from the staff roster, hopefully snuffing out the *omertà* culture that cultivated such a demoralising conspiracy of cheating.

> ❝The Tour is like Formula One… That's why nutrition, training science and gear selection are all on my cycling coaching menu.❞
>
> **Daniel HEALEY,** *Tinkoff Sport*

It's also worth confessing that *The Science of the Tour de France* concentrates on the science-based application of training, nutrition and equipment. The science of a rider's mind and how the rider interacts within the team is a growing field but that's for another time. Of course, that doesn't mean scientists and gear manufacturers have carte blanche to send Froome and Contador to the finish line anyway they'd like. The UCI are known for, at times, what seem like draconian regulations, especially when it comes to bike design, to ensure the sport doesn't become all about the bike. Relevant rules are flagged up throughout the book, and the increasingly innovative methods employed by the bike industry to overcome them.

No other sport pushes the limits like professional cycling. That's why it's such a receptive platform to, as Team Sky winningly term it, 'marginal gains'. Though don't think what you're about to learn is for the elites only. Many of the techniques and practices discussed can easily be transferred to your own performance. Granted, you might not ascend a mountain with the grace of Nairo Quintana or generate the time-trial power of Fabian Cancellara, but that matters not. Apply much of the information that follows – aside perhaps from the 10-grand bikes – to your own performance and you'll become the best cyclist you can be. It might not send you to the podium in Paris but it'll be the price of a book well spent. *Allez, allez, allez…*

 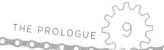

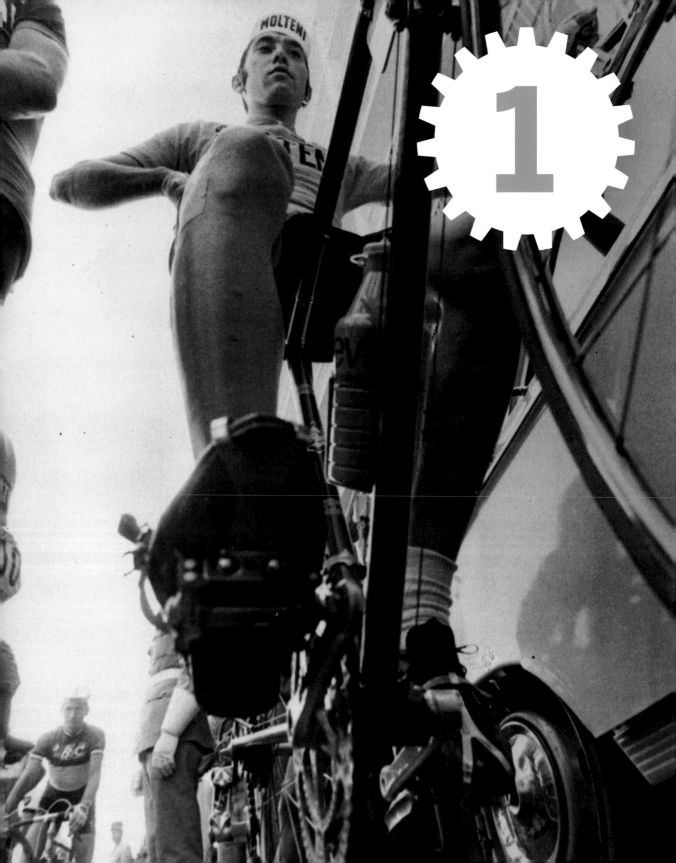

# POWER METERS

## THE BIRTHPLACE OF MODERN CYCLING

'Ride, lots,' Eddy Merckx famously replied when once asked for training advice. Clearly it worked, as the Belgian rider accumulated a palmarès that dominates the test of time: five titles each at the Tour de France and Giro d'Italia, 28 classics, 96 days in the yellow jersey … the list extends to a record 525 victories. Merckx's more-is-more approach certainly paid off. Fellow five-time winner Jacques Anquetil, on the other hand, preferred intensity over huge mileage, two-hour speed sessions behind a car forming the core of his training plan.

Whatever the training approach, effort was measured by a map, stopwatch and beads of sweat, the severity of the ride determined by occasional sprints, racing your teammates and hills. For many, upwards of 400km per week was the norm. As Merckx showed, it worked for some but the advent of training tools offered a more precise method for a rider and team to reach their goals, which has become ever-important in the commercial world of professional cycling. And there's been no greater technological impact on the peloton than the power meter.

'I wish you had invented the SRM when I won the jersey in 1983 in Switzerland. I would have won many more.' The words of three-time Tour de France winner Greg LeMond, hand-written on a rainbow jersey he gifted to SRM power-meter founder Ulrich Schoberer. (SRM takes its name from its inventor, standing for Schoberer Rad Meßtechnik.) In 1986, Schoberer, an engineering student who raced bicycles, sat pondering the inefficiencies of current methods of rider feedback. 'Cadence,

◁ Eddy Merckx during the 1972 Tour de France, which he went onto win for the fourth successive time. He had the power but relied on a stopwatch

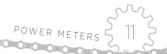

speed and heart rate,' he thought, 'could all be affected by variables such as wind direction, temperature and terrain.' Power output isn't, though, and he set about designing and building the crank-based SRM that hit the market in 1988 (coincidentally LeMond was one of Schoberer's first customers).

For years, the SRM remained the preserve of a few recreational riders and even fewer professionals. Cost and complexity held it back from taking over the masses; for professionals racing in the 1990s, its evolution was stunted by the tip of a needle.

'Doping slowed down the development of scientific techniques to improve performance, and that includes the advancement and integration of power meters,' says Mikel Zabala, sports scientist and coach to Movistar, whose roster includes 2015 Tour de France runner-up Nairo Quintana. 'There were few coaches, no psychologists, no biomechanists … People believed doping was the only thing.

'Now the sport is cleaner and they're at the heart of every rider's training. They help quantify not just the amount of training a rider should do but also training load, their response to training stimulus, making connections between past performances and making predictions for the future. And it can help you change your strategy during races, too.'

For evidence, simply watch Chris Froome's ascent of Mont Ventoux at the 2013 Tour. Over 59 debilitating minutes that ended in stage victory (though followed soon after by a medic strapping an oxygen mask to his face), Froome can be seen regularly glancing down to his SRM. Five times he attacked, each time putting the power down before checking his SRM for the results. He knew his threshold, how long he could max out for and how many times. It worked, of course – he won the first of his two Tours.

## WATT IS POWER?

At its simplest level, power equals force, multiplied by distance, divided by time, and is measured in watts (like your light bulb used to be before lumens came along). In cycling circles it's the energy required to move rider and bike over a certain distance. Calculating the power output of a cyclist is more complex than that but it gives you a rough idea that the more force a cyclist generates, the greater the power, the further they will travel. Strain gauges within a power meter measure this via what is termed a 'balanced electrical circuit'; in other words, resistance is known and constant.

As a force is applied, the shape of the gauge deforms, causing its electrical resistance to alter. There's also the 'piezoelectric effect', which is the voltage generated by squashing electrons. These two reactions to the applied force upset the balance of the circuit, and it's this difference and the resultant electromagnetic force that's effectively being measured and converted into a quantifiable measurement of force. Just remember that if and when the UCI (cycling's national governing body) let TV companies show the riders' power output live during races. As Jens

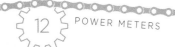

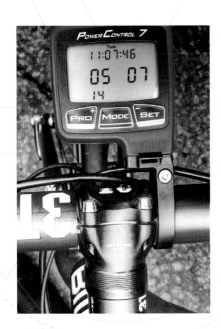

▽ SRM power meter on a BMC bike, Tour de France

Voigt told me, when I caught up with him in England's New Forest just after he'd announced his retirement in 2014, over time you'll see those values rise and rise.

'I remember when I first began racing, I'd push 450 watts for 10 minutes, look back and no one would be with me,' says Voigt, who was known for his daring breakaways. 'Toward the end of my career, I'd do similar and 80 riders would still be with me!'

Schoberer recognised that to accurately calculate the power output of the cyclist, the gauge would have to be as close to the foot's contact point as possible. That's why he integrated his SRM into the cranks. Though not the lightest on the market, it remains the gold standard for measuring power output of cyclists.

'Every rider I know uses power meters now and we still use SRM,' says David Bailey, sports scientist and performance coach at BMC Racing, home to Tejay van Garderen and former hour-record holder Rohan Dennis. 'They're accurate and usable, though there are an increasing number of models hitting the market.'

In 2015, SRM power meters provided metrics for 10 WorldTour teams including Trek-Segafredo, Astana and Tinkoff Sport. Team Sky use Stages, which obtains data from the left crank arm and simply doubles that number for both legs; Ag2r La Mondiale use Quarq; Movistar and Etixx–Quick-Step employ Power2Max; Rotor hook up with Lampre-Merida; Cannondale-Garmin not surprisingly use Garmin's pedal-based Vector; while LottoNL-Jumbo and Giant-Alpecin are powered by Pioneer power meters, which measure power output via both crank arms.

'We used SRM for three years but now we are using Pioneer,' explains Teun van Erp, sports scientist to sprinter John Degenkolb at Giant-Alpecin. 'It's pretty much the same data coming out as SRM so we can transfer historic data to what we're finding from Pioneer.'

Why teams use an increasing range of power meters and not just the original SRM is down to two factors: firstly new meters are now more accurate than rivals to SRM have been in the past, and secondly, sponsorship money talks – it helps fund teams who require a baseline figure of around £7 million per year simply to survive. If your sponsor produces a power meter it's a fair bet you'll adopt it for your team.

Power meters and their use publicly rode into the consciousness of cyclists and cycling fans at the 2012 Tour de France, where Bradley Wiggins and his team, including Chris Froome and Richie Porte, strangled the life out of the opposition by very deliberately riding climbs based on power. There wasn't the romance of 'panache' – the term coined by the French to describe acts of heroism like long breakaways (cue Thomas Voeckler). This was pure, clinical victory by numbers.

# DOWSETT'S EPIPHANY

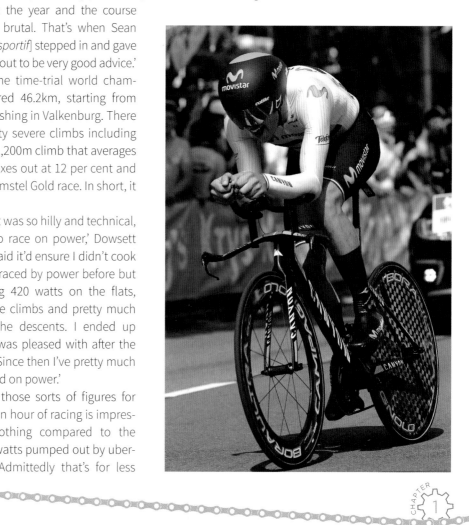

▽ Movistar's Alex Dowsett was converted to the benefits of power meters by his previous employers, Team Sky

Numbers and data are also the domain of time-triallists, for whom every second counts. Movistar's Alex Dowsett, who rode the Tour for the first time in 2015, racked up 52.937km in May that year to briefly hold the hour record, before Bradley Wiggins blew everyone out of the velodrome a month later with 54.526km.

Britain's Dowsett joined Team Sky from Trek-Livestrong's under-23 development team in 2010, before moving to Spanish team Movistar at the end of 2012. Even though he 'just had to get away from Team Sky to do what [he] felt was best for [his] career', Dowsett credits his former employees for switching him onto the potential of power.

'I used to race exclusively on feel,' he remembers. 'In 2012, before I moved to Movistar, I went to the world championships and thought I was going to race pretty badly. I hadn't been performing particularly well after recovering from a broken elbow earlier in the year and the course in Holland was brutal. That's when Sean [Yates, *directeur sportif*] stepped in and gave me what turned out to be very good advice.'

In 2012, the time-trial world championships covered 46.2km, starting from Heerlen and finishing in Valkenburg. There were three pretty severe climbs including the Cauberg, a 1,200m climb that averages 5.8 per cent, maxes out at 12 per cent and features in the Amstel Gold race. In short, it was tough.

'Because it was so hilly and technical, Sean told me to race on power,' Dowsett continues. 'He said it'd ensure I didn't cook myself. I hadn't raced by power before but ended up riding 420 watts on the flats, 450 watts on the climbs and pretty much cruising it on the descents. I ended up eighth, which I was pleased with after the season I'd had. Since then I've pretty much trained and raced on power.'

Averaging those sorts of figures for what was over an hour of racing is impressive, though nothing compared to the reported 1,900 watts pumped out by uber-sprinter Kittel. Admittedly that's for less

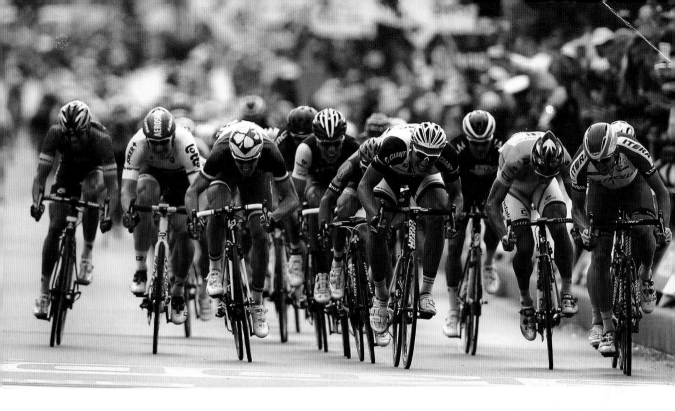

△ Marcel Kittel (centre and then of Giant-Shimano) has reportedly hit 1,900 watts when sprinting to victory

than 10 seconds. Mind you, Kittel wouldn't be aware of the numbers generating beneath him as, like many professional riders, he's known to conceal the power-meter display during racing so the numbers don't distract him from his intuition of when to time the sprint. Balancing power and instinct is a subject picked up on by Movistar's sports scientist Zabala.

'Quintana would make a break on a hill based on both feel and the power meter,' he says, 'but the rider that's depending on power in a race is lost. You need to be creative and hear your feelings. Maybe that's why Nairo or Contador are very brave and attack from far out. In these situations, other riders might think this is suicide. Many of their rivals might look at their power meter and think they can't maintain that wattage. But Nairo looks at their faces, their position in the peloton, at many other variables. To be creative, to be brave, is part of the story.'

So while power meters no doubt have a role to play in races, it's in training that their true worth is measured.

## COMMON TRAINING LANGUAGE

In the 1990s, Chris Boardman's battle with Graeme Obree grew into the stuff of legend. Both men were time-triallists and had dreamt of breaking the hour record set by Italy's Francesco Moser in 1984. The man born of science, Boardman, broke the record on his advanced and very expensive Lotus super-bike constructed from monocoque carbon. Obree, the son of a Scottish policeman, also broke the record, though in more parochial fashion. He used a homemade bike featuring parts from a washing machine.

'Graeme was incredible,' says Boardman, 'and I love the idea of racing and training purely on feel, like Graeme did. But I think, for the most part, those days are numbered.'

While Boardman turned professional, carving out a career with French teams GAN and Crédit Agricole, Obree remained amateur, most recently breaking the world speed record for cycling in the prone position. Boardman retired from professional racing in 2000, and now has his own bike brand as well as commentating annually on the Tour de France for ITV. Boardman was an early adopter of power meters and recognises the impact they've had on the professional peloton today.

'There have been lots of red herrings over the past 20 years, but hidden in the noise are some clever ideas and truths,' he explains in his Liverpudlian twang. 'One of those is power meters, though without knowing what to do with the information, all you had was lots of numbers. That's where Peter Keen [Boardman's coach] came in. He was a much bigger pioneer of power meters than he's even been given credit for because he created a common language for training.'

Keen was one of the first in the country to study the new degree of sports science, at University College Chichester, after representing the national track squad as a junior. In 1986, at the age of just 22, he started working with Boardman. Six years later, Boardman rode to 4,000m pursuit gold at the Barcelona Olympics – Britain's first Olympic cycling gold since 1920. Keen became performance director of British Cycling in 1996, which tied in with the first year of Lottery funding. His influence, Boardman believes, specifically with regard to power training by zones, changed the whole culture of British Cycling and, over time, the direction of professional cycling.

'Keen created training zones for power meters,' says Boardman. 'They were levels one to four, with each focusing on a different physiological improvement. Nowadays that's grown to six or seven depending on the coach but that was a

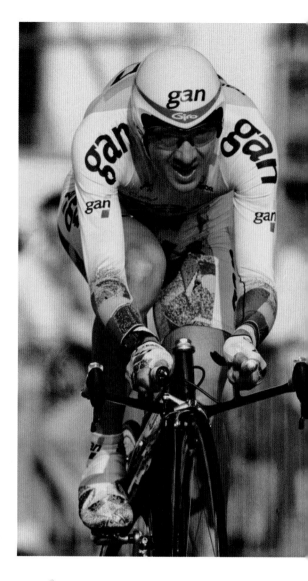

△ Chris Boardman, in his racing days for French team GAN, has always been a fan of power meters

fundamental step forward because it took out the emotional descriptive measurement of effort, which had simply been "really hard", "really easy"… which obviously mean different things to different people.'

Keen's employment of power and training zones complemented two further training measurements – heart rate and the rider's feedback of task difficulty. 'The three Ps,' as Boardman calls them – power, pulse and perception – ignited a cycling revolution that eventually saw Dave Brailsford, who'd been working with British Cycling on a consultancy basis since 1998, become Performance Director in 2003 following Keen's departure. Brailsford and British Cycling continued Keen's good work, maximising the three Ps and helping the team to win two more golds at the 2004 Olympics before GB ramped that up to eight golds each in Beijing and London. In the meantime, Brailsford launched and became manager of Team Sky in 2010, overseeing both Wiggins' and Froome's victories in the 2012, 2013 and 2015 editions of the Tour de France.

'Where power is now at Team Sky and elsewhere is down to Keen,' Boardman says. 'Team Sky basically copied British Cycling and the work started by Keen.'

As Boardman alluded to, many WorldTour teams now employ the seven-zone system devised by the American Dr Andrew Coggan and Hunter Allen, which was an evolution of Keen's work. There's more detail on the different aims of each zone in the 'Training by numbers' box (see page 18) but, briefly, Coggan's categories are (in order of intensity): active recovery, endurance, tempo, lactate threshold, $VO_2$ max, anaerobic capacity and neuromuscular power. Their use is situation specific but the active recovery zone, for instance, would be used after strenuous training days or races.

In days gone by, cyclists' training plans comprised a bottle of water and the soigneur yelling at the rider to '*allez, allez, allez*', usually until the sun had set and the rider had turned a ghostly pale. Now, the majority of professional riders' training plans are based on zones.

'The power meter and prescriptive zones have certainly changed the way I approach training,' says American Brent Bookwalter, who races for BMC Racing and has completed the Tour three times. 'At any given time in the year, we're following different training zones and ticking off the session, though it's interesting that because we've racked up so many miles, many of us could probably self-prescribe these intensities and come close to what the power meter would say. But there's so much riding on the Tour these days that it's good to be accountable.'

# THE RENAISSANCE GUY

Daniel Healey is the former head of sports science at Tinkoff Sport. Healey moved from BMC Racing at the end of 2014 in a move that reflected the increasingly important role sports science is playing in professional cycling. 'I've been using SRMs and training zones since my university days back in the mid-90s,' says the

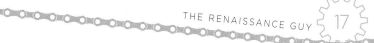

# Training by numbers

○ **American coaches Dr Andrew Coggan and Hunter Allen** developed the following seven-zone system of power training for riders to work more accurately on certain physiological and performance parameters. Often, professional teams will have these zones and individual wattage ranges taped to the riders' stems on training rides.

| TRAINING ZONE | POWER OUTPUT | PHYSIOLOGICAL ADAPTATION | PERFORMANCE BENEFIT |
|---|---|---|---|
| 1 Recover | < 55% of threshold | Increases blood flow to flush out waste products and deliver nutrients | Boosts recovery; lays foundation for harder sessions |
| 2 Base endurance | 56–75% | Stimulates fat metabolism; prepares muscles, tendons, ligaments and nervous system for cycling | More efficient use of energy |
| 3 Tempo | 76–90% | Boosts carbohydrate metabolism; changes some slow-twitch muscles to fast-twitchers | Increases sustainable power |
| 4 Threshold | 91–105% | Further boosts ability to metabolise carbohydrate; develops lactate threshold | Improves sustainable race pace, though too much time in this zone can cause staleness and fatigue |
| 5 Maximal aerobic power | 106–120% | Builds cardiovascular system and VO$_2$ max | Improves time-trialling ability and resistance to short-term fatigue |
| 6 Anaerobic capacity | >121% | Short, intense efforts of 30 seconds to 3 minutes increase anaerobic capacity | Builds the ability to break from the group |
| 7 Neuromuscular power | Maximal | Raises maximum muscle power; develops neural control of pedalling at specific cadence | Good for short sprints |

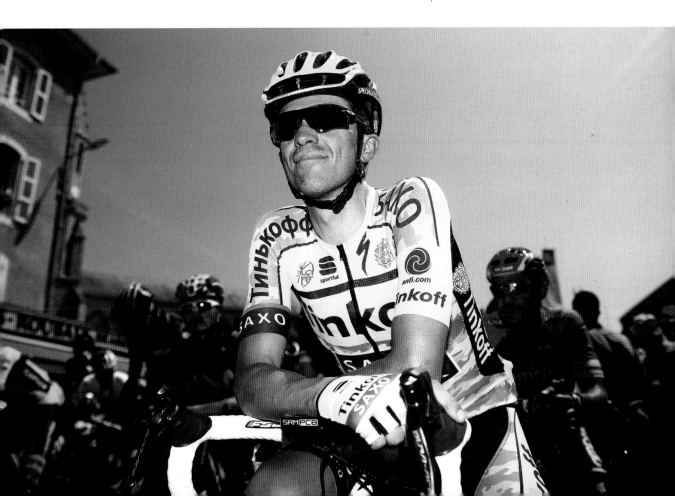

New Zealander. 'It's ironic because back then I wouldn't have been able to get the job I had at Tinkoff – they simply didn't exist in professional cycling.'

Healey is a renaissance man of sports science, his expertise stretching from coaching to nutrition, physiology to equipment. It's his 'intellectual property' that had billionaire owner Oleg Tinkov flashing his credit card once more in pursuit of victory.

'I'll give you an example of how zones work,' says Healey. 'In December, for a guy like Alberto [Contador], we were already specifically building to the Tour de France in July. By that I mean we were making him fit and then strong, but not doing too much power work or high intensity. What we know with confidence is that training within certain training zones will produce a series of physiological modifications that will set up a rider like Alberto for a long and successful season.'

During December, in general the aim is to build a strong base that'll lay the foundations for more intense work once the echoes of Auld Lang Syne have died down and race season approaches – which is as early as January and the Tour Down Under for many riders.

The early-season modifications Healey cited primarily focus on improving a rider's capacity to transport and utilise oxygen – nectar when it comes to ultra-endurance events like the Tour de France. These adaptations are numerous but five

▽ Like nearly all professionals, Spain's Alberto Contador trains by power zones

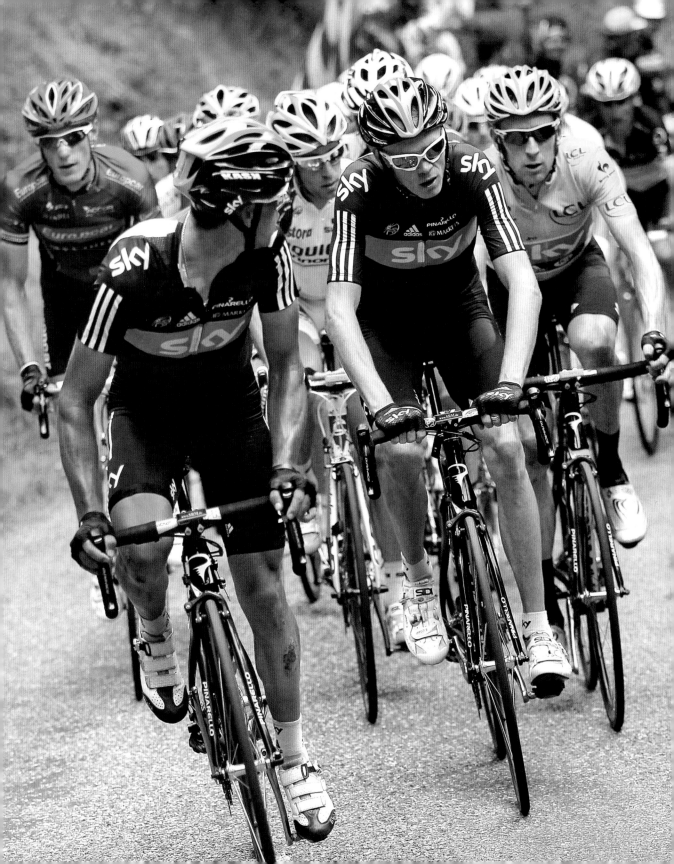

of the most significant are: increasing the number of mitochondria in the exercising muscles; increasing the size and number of muscle capillaries; increasing haemoglobin and blood plasma levels to enhance oxygen transport; better thermoregulation due to increased plasma volume and improved circulation; and greater glycogen storage, which becomes useful for higher-intensity race efforts down the line. 'To achieve this, we'd instruct our riders to target recovery or high tempo wattages [but still relatively low intensity] for most of November and December,' adds Healey.

Which is all well and good but how do Healey and Kerrison at Team Sky set training zones like active recovery and tempo? 'We profile each and every rider during the off-season training camps and test them not only to see if their fitness is improving but also to set the individual training zones for each rider,' explains Healey.

'To set each zone, we need a centrepiece to work from and this is what we call "threshold". One definition is the maximum power you can hold for one hour, though that can be quite tiring and affect the gains you're looking for in subsequent training sessions, so we tend to feature this at the end of training camps and keep it to 20 minutes. With that number, we slice off 5 per cent to give an hour's prediction and a threshold figure.'

# IMPORTANCE OF THRESHOLD

The reason threshold or lactate threshold is chosen as the yardstick by which all other zones are set is because it's the most important physiological determinant of endurance cycling performance, since it integrates three key variables: $VO_2$ max, the percentage of $VO_2$ max that can be sustained for a given duration and cycling efficiency.

'Basically, threshold is the point where you're consuming as much lactic acid as you are producing,' adds Healey. 'You can recycle much of it and sit on that uncomfortable level for a long time. Above that and lactate starts to accumulate and that's where we hit the red zones, or $VO_2$ zone. There's only so much work you should do in those and you should only do that work in controlled doses, though essentially the higher the threshold, the stronger the rider.'

A professional rider's functional threshold (functional threshold and threshold are interchangeable terms when it comes to power) is a guarded secret, though Bradley Wiggins has been reported to have a functional threshold of between 440 and 460 watts, which helped him sustain the pace to smash the hour record, whereas a leaked photo at the 2015 Tour reportedly showed Alberto Contador's at 420 watts. A good recreational rider, who trains for about five to seven hours each week, would be below 250 watts. In fact, so important is threshold and power data to a rider's performance that Team Sky released to French newspaper *L'Équipe* two years' worth of Chris Froome's power data in light of drug speculation at the 2013 Tour. (Experts

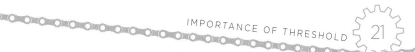

concluded that Froome's power dips of around 60 watts over intense one-hour efforts were what you'd expect of a clean rider as the Tour progresses.) They felt compelled to do similar at the 2015 Tour, which we examine in the 'Froome power' box.

Once each rider's individual zones have been calculated, it's common for the coaches to print out the zones on a piece of card and stick them to the rider's stem. 'That's something I brought to the team,' says Healey. 'There's a grey line running right across the middle of the card and that's where threshold sits. During early winter, we'd tell the riders to train below that middle line. If they go over it, it is not the training adaptation we are after.'

Much of what Healey and his brethren apply with regard to training zones and specific training sessions is clearly a competitive advantage, so the preserve of meetings not media, though Healey is generous enough to reveal a power-based session that Tinkoff Sport riders would undertake during the winter months.

'One session that's stood the test of time is the two-phase hill repeats, which is simply a hill that's ridden at two distinctly different intensities. Used concurrently with specific strength work, we use this session when a rider's in their base phase.

'The rider will enter the hill at endurance wattage, then continue at the same intensity for the first half of the climb. At the mid-point of the two-phase hill, the rider will switch up to a higher intensity (somewhere in their tempo zone – 266 to 318 watts, for instance) and hold this all the way to the crest of the climb.'

Healey says that over a four-week block of training, the riders might complete these efforts twice a week with a progressive overload that might begin at something like four of these two-hill reps inside a longer ride of 3–4 hours at endurance/tempo wattage. By week three, the number of reps might have doubled to eight over a 5-hour ride, but holding the same intensity.

## Froome power

○ The 2015 Tour de France was dominated by Chris Froome and Team Sky – so much so that speculation of doping predictably grew into the overriding narrative among many pundits and ex-racers. In an attempt to diffuse the situation, the team released some of Froome's power data from stage 10, where the Brit took a stranglehold on the race, specifically the 15.3km climb to the finish at La Pierre-Saint-Martin.

Head of Athlete Performance Tim Kerrison told the press conference, 'We have a lot of data on our riders and the way we apply and use it, we see that gives us a competitive advantage. As in most industries, knowledge and intelligence is giving a competitive advantage.

'It's difficult to indicate the exact start of the climb,' he continued, 'so I've analysed the last 15.3km, which is an effort of about 41 and a half minutes.'

Kerrison revealed that Froome's average power output came in at 414 watts for the 41 minutes 28 seconds of effort. Froome's functional threshold – the wattage he can maintain for one hour – isn't known but examining his contemporaries' one-hour figures (Sir Bradley Wiggins' reported threshold is 440–460 watts) suggests Froome's figure is plausible.

What confused many was Froome's power-to-weight ratio. (We discuss power-to-weight in detail in Chapter 8.) This came in at 6.13 watts per kilogramme but Sky corrected this to 5.78 to allow for over-reporting of power when using elliptical chainrings, as used by Froome.

Sports scientist Ross Tucker has analysed power outputs over the years on his Sports Science website. He questioned those figures, suggesting Froome couldn't have ridden so fast at that power output.

'However, I think there are two ways that those figures can be justified and a combination of the two explains it for me,' he commented on his website at the time. 'The manufacturer [of the chainrings] claims 4 per cent [as the correct reduction to compensate for over-reporting of power] but Tim Kerrison reduces the measured power output by 6 per cent. I think if they reduced it by 4 per cent, then the power output they would have got would have been higher. Not a lot higher, but enough.

'414 watts is what is produced on the reading. So if you knock 414 down by 6 per cent, you get 389. What they have then done is divided that by 67.5kg [Froome's weight] and they get 5.77. But if you put in that 414 and brought it down by 4 per cent, then what you get is 397. That translates to 5.89 watts per kilo on that same mass.'

Tucker then goes on to suggest that if Froome's pre-Dauphiné weight (the race Froome won in June) of 66kg is used instead of the 67.5kg, you end up with 6.02 watts per kilogram: 'it starts to add up'.

In August, Froome headed to the GSK Human Performance Lab in London to begin a series of physiological tests to prove his performance was based on natural, rather than illegal, means.

The results went public in December 2015 and showed that Froome has a peak power of 525 watts and sustained power of 419 watts for between 20-40 minutes. His $VO_2$ max came in at 84.6ml/kg. All three parameters of performance showed no suspicion of doping. Instead, his improvement from his last recorded physiological test in 2007 was deemed to be down to weight loss. In 2007 he weighed 75.6kg; at the 2015 Tour he measured just 67kg.

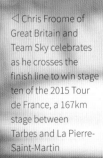

◁ Chris Froome of Great Britain and Team Sky celebrates as he crosses the finish line to win stage ten of the 2015 Tour de France, a 167km stage between Tarbes and La Pierre-Saint-Martin

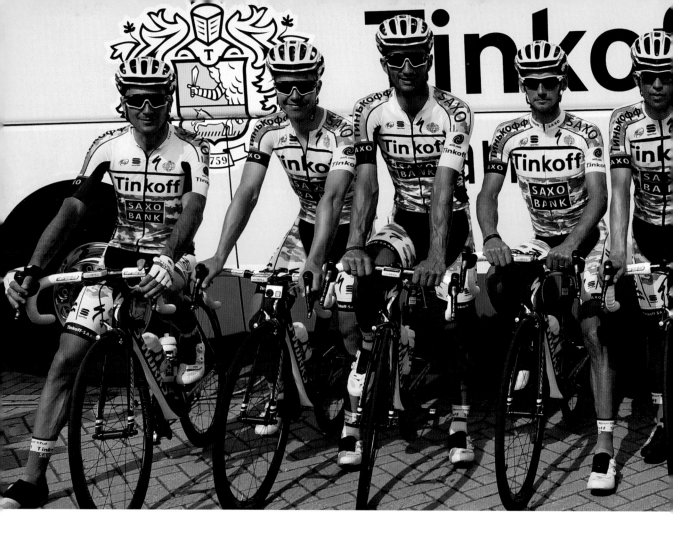

## ANALYSING THE RESULTS

Of course, it's one thing setting zones – it's another monitoring that the riders aren't taking it easy (unusual) or going too hard (common). 'After every training ride, we upload our data for the coaches to analyse,' says Trek-Segafredo's Bauke Mollema, who finished seventh at the 2015 Tour de France. 'It's good because you and the coaches can compare data to the previous month or previous week.'

The advent of wireless technology means information from the power meter can be uploaded to a computer or mobile phone in seconds, but with no analytical tool to examine and interpret the data, the rider would be all dressed up with nowhere to go. 'We're supported by TrainingPeaks and that's the software that every rider uploads their training to,' says BMC's coach David Bailey. 'Now we have a policy on the team that if the riders don't do that, they will not race.'

TrainingPeaks is an online analysis software package that, it could be argued,

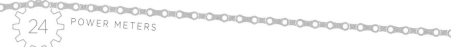

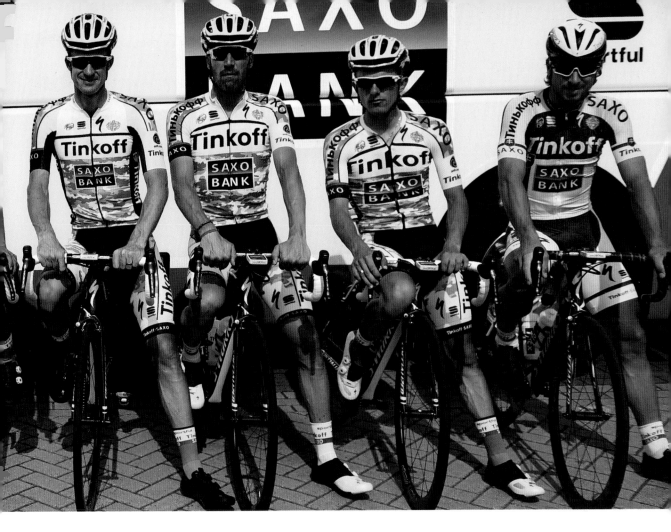

△ Tinkoff Sport riders, including Alberto Contador, use SRM power meters

is why so many teams now rely on wattage. 'In the past, we'd have had to use a pen and paper and note down figures,' says Boardman. 'Now it is much more accessible and nowhere near as complex.'

TrainingPeaks is the brainchild of Dirk Friel, son of famous American coach Joe, and Gear Fisher, an engineer and cyclist. 'We created TrainingPeaks back in 1999 and went live in 2000,' explains Friel. 'The first customers were triathletes but we had our cycling breakthrough in 2007 – the year that Bob Stapleton took over at T-Mobile. He wanted more accountability and a clean sport. Under Bob we worked with the team and then started working with the Belgium team Lotto.

'The following year we started working with Saxo, and that's proved our longest partnership,' Friel continues. 'We haven't skipped a beat since 2008. [Coach] Bobby Julich brought us into Saxo and then he moved to Sky, then BMC, then went back to Saxo, so went full circle. And then, in his second year with Team Sky, Tim Kerrison reached out to us to start leveraging our system.'

TrainingPeaks creates a series of graphs that plot factors like how the rider's power output fluctuates over the course of a training ride or race. You can then compare this day-by-day, week-by-week, to see if the training is having the desired effect: to race longer and faster. Probably the greatest development has been in managing fatigue and form to peak for races but, says Friel, its key sell is flexibility.

'There's no one proper way to use our system,' he says. 'Each team and each coach has a different methodology and their own metrics and data points that they're looking at each day. Some teams, a coach will be looking at each individual stage file of the Tour and gaining feedback from that. Did the rider hit any peak power values today? How hard was the stage? What was the stress score of the day? How does that relate to previous stages? Where should the athlete be at this point in a stage race? Are they at a fatigue level where they can perform five days from now at the major climbs?

'Certain coaches look at every data file, every day, and then they can turn around and discuss that with the *directeur sportif*,' Friel continues. 'The conversation might be along the lines of, "They'll be ready to go four days from now." Or, "Don't push them too hard tomorrow – hold them back." This feeds back into the potential strategy for an upcoming stage.'

▽ Bradley Wiggins chats to team coach Shane Sutton as they take a break during a training ride in Les Herbiers, France

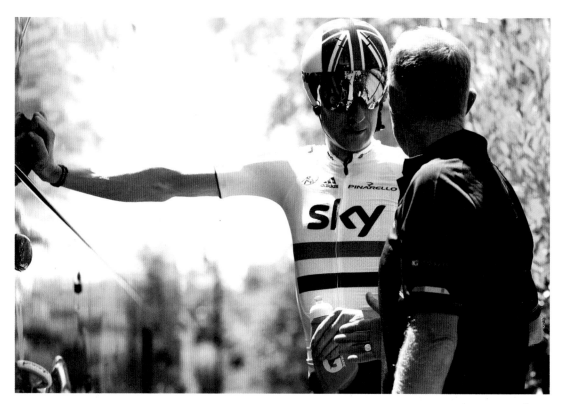

# ROGERS'S STAGE VICTORY

Another benefit of TrainingPeaks is giving the wider audience an insight into a professional rider's day, revealing aspects like how many watts they push up huge climbs, how fast they ride and how many calories they burn. Take the 2014 Tour de France as an example.

TrainingPeaks, with permission from the teams, published files from every single day of the 21 stages. Tinkoff Sport's Michael Rogers downloaded his data for the Grand Départ from Leeds to Harrogate. Over the 190km stage, hidden in a graph that looks like an ECG profile, you could observe that Rogers burnt 4,007 calories and held 445 watts for 11 minutes and 23 seconds on the first climb. Come the second climb that had dropped to 388 watts for just over 8 minutes. The data also showed Rogers pedalled with an unusually low cadence for the stage – 79rpm. The next day, the 201km stage from York to Sheffield, Rogers burned 4,860 calories during the five-and-a-half hour stage and during the Cote de Holme Moss climb averaged 361 watts. For the entire stage, he averaged 319 watts.

This data is automatically sent to the coach's mobile phone for analysis, and you can see how the team begins to paint an accurate picture of a rider's form and nutritional requirements. Rogers continued to send his files to TrainingPeaks for use and publication. Stage 15 – 222km from Tallard to Nîmes – was one of the windiest and wettest days of the 2014 Tour. Rogers burned 800 calories an hour for over five hours, averaged 336 watts for the final hectic hour before generating a peak 30-second effort of 634 watts with just 5km to go. That's some effort at the end of a long stage, but not enough to prevent Katusha's Alexander Kristoff from taking the honours.

Despite a debilitating day in the saddle, that night Rogers and his team examined the data and knew he had form. 'We had stage 16 in mind and the team were right behind me,' says Rogers. 'It was the longest stage of the Tour but it was the last opportunity where the leading teams would let the riders go who weren't in contention.'

Rogers formed part of a 21-man breakaway that soon carved out a 10-minute lead over the peloton. Twenty-one had shrunk to five come the peak of the day's biggest climb, the Port de Balès, with Rogers lining up beside Sky's Vasil Kiryienka, Lampre-Merida's José Serpa, and Europcar's Thomas Voeckler and Cyril Gautier.

The stage seemed set up for French team Europcar to deliver glory to sprinter Gautier, but Rogers surprised all by attacking with over 4km to go. Gautier, caught off guard, couldn't catch Rogers's rear wheel and the former Australian national pursuit champion used all his years of experience to take his first-ever stage victory at the Tour.

'In hindsight it was a bit of a suicide mission,' explains Rogers. 'It was a bit cat-and-mouse but I didn't want to go too hard in that initial break because no one would come with you. And no one wants to ride 200km on their own. I was the only one present from my team whereas Europcar had a couple of riders. I've been around long enough to know that when you see the chances arrive, you must take them.'

Though he admits he didn't make that race-winning break by power alone, his files showed (see the 'Power profile' box below) that after being in the break for six hours, Rogers held an average power output of 377 watts for the final 4 minutes 35 seconds and averaged 35mph. He'd also burnt 6,639 calories. Though Rogers might not have been sprinting by numbers, you can guarantee that the coach would have known Rogers's chances of stage victory rested on his individual pursuit past. They looked at the TrainingPeaks data on stage 15, could see he'd have the power to lead a break and, though he was no sprinter, would retain a high wattage for the not inconsiderable length of 4km.

'As Michael showed, TrainingPeaks is a really useful tool, though I also have my own spreadsheets of power data stacked up from the years,' says Healey. 'Through the season, the rider receives detailed feedback every Sunday night or Monday morning, which is a summary of the week just gone by. It's held up against the template for each rider's development and then we base the upcoming week against that data. That's how it works.'

Though TrainingPeaks is the software used by the majority of teams, including Team Sky and Movistar, it's not the only software around. BMC's Bailey flags up a programme called Golden Cheetah that he sees as equally impressive. 'It has been developed by Phil Skiba, who used to work at Exeter University (England) and is an MIT graduate from the US,' says Bailey. 'He created software and algorithms based on research he did that involved getting a load of guys to exercise in an MRI and examining the depletion of phosphates. Phosphates give you energy, whether it's during aerobic exercise when you have oxygen or down to your most immediate energy system,

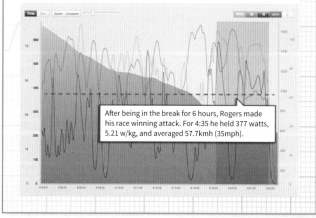

## Power profile

○ TrainingPeaks software shows the power output generated by Tinkoff Sport's Michael Rogers en route to winning stage 16 of the 2014 Tour de France. Rogers's wattage profile is illustrated in pink. TrainingPeaks also shows his speed (in km/h, green) and cadence (rpm, orange).

**Stage 16 – Carcassonne to Bagenéres-de-Luchon – 237.5km**
Michael Rogers (Team Tinkoff Saxo)

After being in the break for 6 hours, Rogers made his race winning attack. For 4:35 he held 377 watts, 5.21 w/kg, and averaged 57.7kmh (35mph).

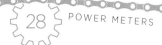

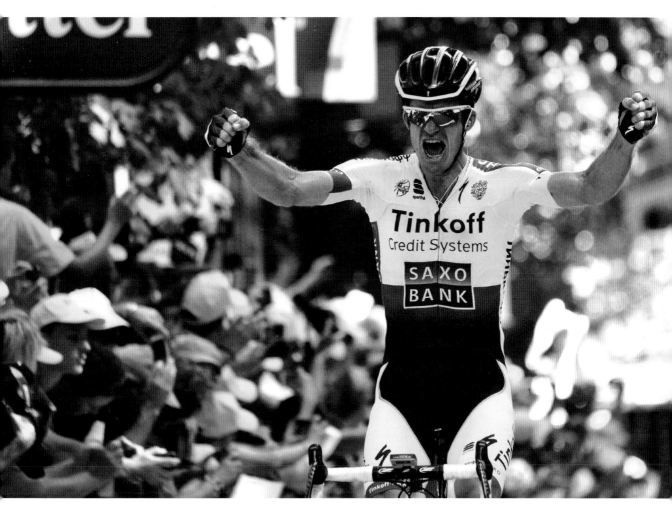

△ Australia's Michael Rogers combined power data and intuition to win the 16th stage of the 2014 Tour de France

the ATP-PC system, that supplies you with 8–10 seconds of energy. He could observe how they're depleted and replenished by asking the guys to ride at high intensity and then recover at different intensities at or below threshold. With that data, he created a mathematical model that helped to devise training zones for all riders – without them having to have an MRI scan.'

Whether teams remain with TrainingPeaks, leap onto Golden Cheetah or choose some other power-based software, the fact coaches can calculate what wattages are needed to win certain stages, lead over the stiffest of climbs or create a breakaway means they can take the guesswork out of things. They have a goal figure. They just need to design the right training sessions, manage fatigue and consume the right nutrition, each of which we'll examine in the chapters to follow.

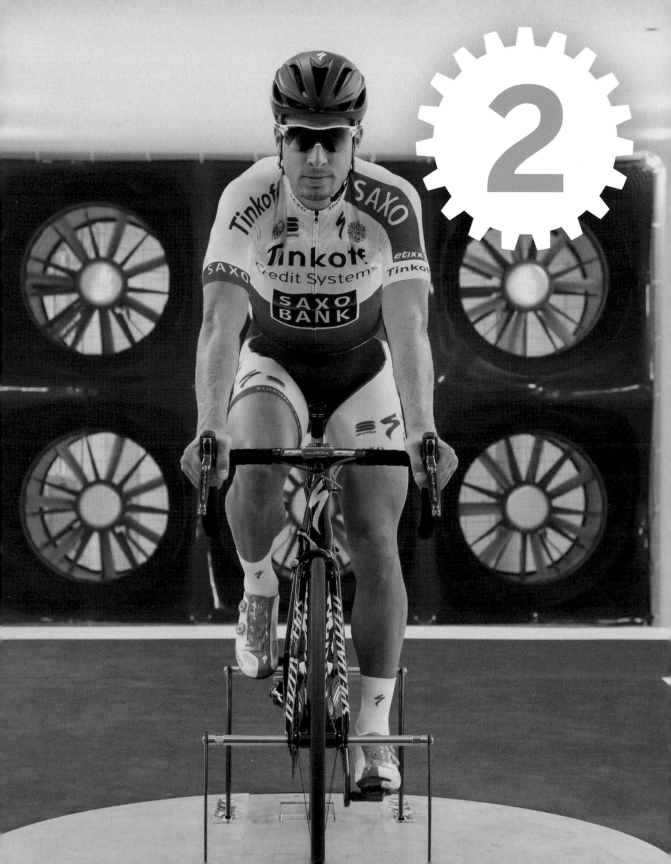

# BIKE FITTING

## POSITION, PREPARE, PERFORM

In *A Sunday In Hell,* the film that centres on the 1976 chapter of Paris–Roubaix and is widely acclaimed as one of the finest pieces of cycling cinematography, two scenes capture five-time Tour de France winner Eddy Merckx's obsession with bike position. On the eve of the cobbled classic, Merckx is shown in the team's hotel triple-checking the position of his saddle and brake levers. It's not long before out comes the spirit level, tape measure and long metal ruler. The next morning, the race is halted by a demonstration. Merckx sees this as an opportunity to roll over to a rival team's car, borrow a spanner and tinker with his saddle once more.

Merckx preceded the world of marginal gains, seeking every competitive advantage to dominate his contemporaries. But Merckx primarily based his changes, his advances, on instinct – which was clearly finely honed as he won over 500 times in a professional career that will probably never be bettered. But with his innovative ideas, surely Merckx would have delighted in the empirical-based technology and accuracy that is WorldTour bike-fitting.

'When I moved from Belkin at the end of 2014, the first thing that Trek [Factory Racing] did was assess my bike position,' says Netherlands' Bauke Mollema, who was the team's GC contender at the 2015 Tour and finished a creditable seventh. 'It was a highly technical and involved process where Cyclefit looked at my body and biomechanics. I appreciated it as, how can I put it, my position on the bike isn't that fluid!'

London-based Cyclefit have been Trek-Segafredo's technical fit partners since

◁ Tinkoff's Peter Sagan, undertaking wind tunnel testing at Specialized's HQ

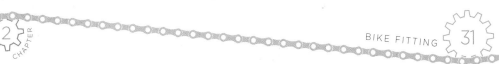

2012. Cyclefit began life in 2001, offering high-tech solutions to the most important interaction – that between rider and bike.

'Generally we'll work with the team at training camps,' says bike-fitter and co-founder Julian Wall. 'It usually pans out that we'll work with the riders over a two-week training camp in Calpe, Spain, before Christmas, another week there in January and then, for some, straight after the Tour of Lombardy in October.'

Like all teams, positional changes happen over the off-season – 'riders won't want to try anything new during the race season' – and it's quite a logistical issue. Cyclefit transfer their London service to wherever Trek-Segafredo are headed, which means shipping their cutting-edge equipment to a destination that's less than salubrious.

'We tend to take over a hotel's basement,' says Wall. 'Thankfully it's not too bad and can often be a conference centre. We'll examine nearly 30 riders with our practitioners looking at bike fit, saddle pressure, flexibility … It's a dynamic, frantic, but organised environment.'

The aim of the bike fit is to make each and every cyclist more efficient. You might think that professionals have naturally 'grown' into their optimum position but even the subtlest of changes can impact on performance. Research from Spain shows that a variance of 0.5cm–1.5cm from optimal saddle position can result in significantly greater energy expenditure. Over 2,000-plus miles, it could be the difference between *le maillot jaune* or *la flamme rouge*.

# THREE KEY CONNECTING POINTS

To unravel the optimum bike position for Fabian Cancellara and co. at Trek, Cyclefit begin with a physical examination. No rubber gloves required – more a physio-led general manipulation of limbs to assess flexibility, range of motion, strengths and weaknesses. The riders then mount a Fit Bike, a stationary structure with movable parts, resembling a bike at the contact points of saddle, handlebars and pedals at least. This is key to the process as Cyclefit can easily manoeuvre the rider without having to dismount and unclip through every iteration.

'It's where we examine the rider's pedal stroke, looking at factors like how their legs extend and what their posture's like,' explains Wall. 'To simplify things, we're looking at three key connecting points in space – the handlebars, saddle and pedals – and can then tweak those on the Fit Bike. Hands, bum and feet are key.'

Wall compares it to being measured for a bespoke suit. Custom bike-fitting is common across all of the Tour teams, though many use Retül, including Tinkoff Sport, Astana and Etixx–Quick-Step – which is hardly surprising as the bike suppliers for those teams, Specialized, bought Retül in 2012.

'We use Retül, too,' says Jonathan Baker, coach for the first African-registered team to race the Tour de France, Team Dimension Data. 'The team were on Trek

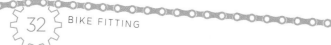

bikes in 2014 but moved to Cervélo at the end of that year. We took their measurements on the Trek and found them similar-sized bikes, and then did Retül bike fits on their bikes to find their optimum position.'

In essence, both Cyclefit and Retül perform the same role. They put the rider into what's deemed optimum position, both spewing out reams of data that are meaningless to laymen but vital for practitioners.

'Of course, it's nice to have the technology, but you need the experience to assimilate and apply that information, especially as many riders are resistant to change,' says Phil Cavell, co-founder with Julian Wall of Cyclefit and a bike-fitter. 'You'll make a tweak and then when you see them again, they've reverted to their old position and are still complaining about the same issues. But as long as you have numbers, you can argue your side; when they see the technology is helping them, that's when hopefully they'll subscribe to what you're doing.'

That technology includes the Fit Bike, which is wired into a Computrainer. This provides variable resistance and works in sync with Spinscan – a package that shows the technician where the power is applied during the pedal stroke and which leg is doing the most work. All of this is filmed by a number of cameras, from the side and face on, to record a full picture of rider and bike. Cyclefit employs a motion-capture system called Dartfish, which measures leg extension and charts key points of movement for analysis during and after the fit. The tracking of the knee is key so lasers are also used to check for lateral movement through the pedal stroke. In fact, a study revealed 23 per cent of injuries suffered by professional cyclists are in the knee.

'The knee is the area that suffers the most as it's sandwiched between foot and bum,' says Wall, 'so we'll adjust the bike to recommended parameters and add an internal footbed [extra insole] to see if that helps. We can add cleats as well if needed but, in all honesty, you want to keep changes to a minimum. At the end of the day, they wouldn't have reached professional status if they constantly pedalled with a dangerously injury-susceptible stroke.'

Specialized bike-fitter Sean Madsen, who's worked with riders of the calibre of Mark Cavendish, suggests otherwise. 'Yes, most of the changes are subtle but every now and then you'll do something more major,' he says. 'It'll often be because they've moved teams or come up from Continental level. I have a saying: all of these riders have Ferrari motors but some are in a Volkswagen body.

'When we were at the Tinkoff-Saxo camp before Christmas 2014, we had to make some pretty significant changes to Edward Beltran,' Madsen continues. 'He'd been experiencing unilateral saddle sores on one side, and we discovered it was all driven by a tibial length inequality of around 5mm. So we put a bit of support and cleat on his short side so he didn't have to reach so far. It helped even him out.'

At a bike-fitting session, the rider's weight distribution on the saddle will be analysed, in the case of Cyclefit via a pressure-mapping tool from German company gebioMized. This tool becomes even more important if the practitioners have tweaked the rider's set-up because adjustments to saddle height can change the orientation on the saddle, so via some rather colourful on-screen patterning, the team can see if there any hotspots.

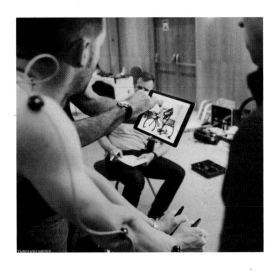

△▷ Ivan Basso, now retired, undergoing 21st-century bike fitting

# RESTRAINED BY THE RULEBOOK

Most of the changes are subtle but there are times when situations demand a more thorough overhaul. 'When the team moved to the new Speed Concept bike, that's when we made the biggest changes,' explains Cavell. 'The riders were very traditional and would always use longer cranks on their time-trial bike. Historically, "experts" said they helped to generate more power. But the power meters don't say that. Many riders have different crank lengths between their road and time-trial bikes. In Fabian's case, this was 175mm for the road and 177.5mm for time trial. The problem is, when you have a very low position, a long crank can prevent you from smoothly moving over the top of the pedal stroke and so limit power.'

Cancellara remained resistant to the changes for two years – not surprising for a man who's won his national time-trial title a record nine times – but is now more receptive. Like his countryman Roger Federer, as Spartacus has grown older, he's had to adapt. 'As you age, you just can't survive on brute strength like the younger lads do,' says Wall. 'Cancellara has great handling skills and tactical acumen for a race like the Tour of Flanders, but in a time trial it's more about harnessing power.'

Cancellara's also hamstrung by UCI (Union Cycliste Internationale) rules that stipulate the peak of a rider's saddle can't be further back than 5cm lateral of the bottom bracket. The rule was brought in to prevent extreme positions like those seen

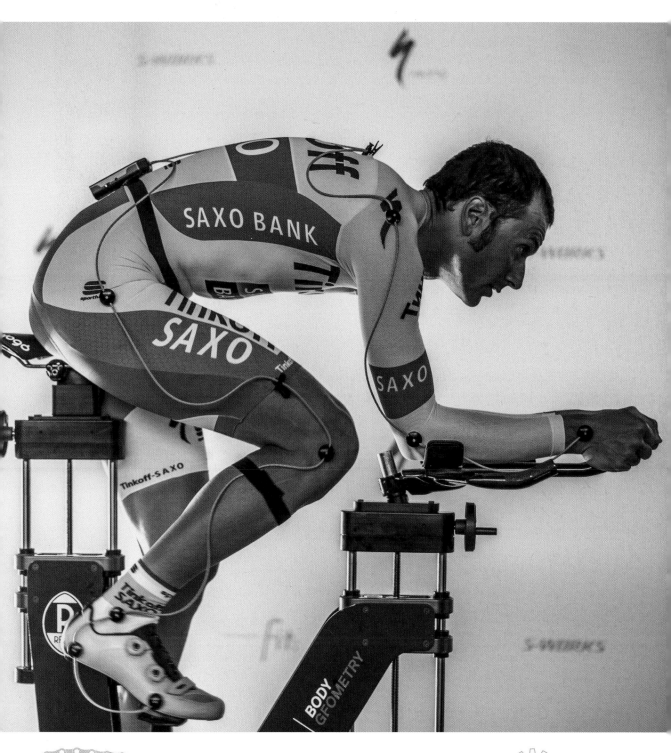

in the early 1990s by Messrs Boardman and Obree. 'That's all very well but Fabian's 6ft 2in,' says Wall. 'He has an 85cm reach to the bars but, if he was allowed, could probably go up to 90cm. He'd go quicker if he had more space to express himself.'

During the time-trial makeover, Cyclefit also raised many of the riders' bars slightly so they were closer to their road position. 'You lose 30–40 watts from road to time trial when going super-aero,' says Wall. 'That tweak was designed to limit those losses.'

# RIDE LIKE THE WIND

Bike fit is just one factor in the positional equation. As well as bike manufacturers spending thousands on wind-tunnel time in search of slipstreaming frames and forks, teams send riders in, too. It's the next step in position optimisation.

'In a time trial, at high speeds – say 45km/h – you're looking at around 85 per cent drag from the person and 15 per cent from the bike,' says aerodynamicist Simon Smart. 'Someone who's optimised their position on the bike can redress that to more like 65–35.'

In 2014, Smart, who's also the brains behind Enve wheels and the Scott Plasma bike, began testing the Movistar team in the UK-based wind-tunnel he uses with his company Drag2Zero, to impressive results. Alejandro Valverde won the Spanish time-trial national championships for the first time; Nairo Quintana had one of his best-ever time trials en route to winning the Giro d'Italia; and Adriano Malori won the time trial on the last day of the 2014 Vuelta.

'It's all little details with the elite; about understanding which element of position gives efficiency,' says a modest Smart, before highlighting the increased role aerodynamics plays in professional cycling. 'When I started the company, we primarily had the time-triallists in but now so many Grand Tours are being decided by time trials that we're having GC riders in, too. Riders are becoming more interested in aerodynamics and cutting their Cd.'

Cd is the rider's *coefficient of drag* and is key to helping aerodynamicists like Smart make their subjects more streamlined and, in turn, ride faster. *Aerodynamic drag* is air resistance attributed to an object. That figure is a product of an object's drag coefficient (Cd), or 'slippiness', and its size – in particular, its frontal area (A). Drag is simply those two figures multiplied.

The coefficient of aerodynamic drag (CdA) ranges upwards of zero. Physics dictates that an object with a drag coefficient of zero can't exist on Earth – everything that exists, however streamlined, has some drag. But the numbers can be satisfyingly low – teardrop-shaped handlebars on a top-end bike can register a figure of 0.005. (We discuss teardrop shapes and their aerodynamic impact in more detail in Chapter 5.) That's aero. A brick might be 2.0. Unsurprisingly, that's not aero. CdA examples of elite riders using aero-shaped bars might come in at the 0.18–0.25 mark.

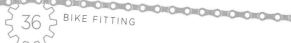

# What is drag?

○ It's the bane of a cyclist's life that drag increases the faster you go. How does that work, you might ask? Well, it's a touch complex but bear with me.

Air pressure creates a force that's proportional to the square of the rider's speed. Added to this, the power to propel the cyclist through the air increases as the cube of velocity. In essence, this means that going twice as fast requires eight times the power. It's been shown that Tour riders will expend 90 per cent of their energy overcoming air pressure as they hit speeds of 54km/h, unless they're drafting in a pack.

Drag is influenced by many factors including shape, texture and boundary layer separation (essentially how quickly a layer of air leaves the tubing and causes turbulence), and is why reducing frontal profile is the aim of all riders. This can include things like tucking the elbows in slightly and keeping that teardrop-shaped aero helmet in line with the back.

This image of a time-triallist from one of Cervelo's CFD (computational fluid dynamics) technicians highlights how drag varies throughout the body. The colours on the surface indicate pressure, with high pressure shown in red and low pressure in blue. You can see how even tweaking your hand position to a more acute angle, so there's a smaller frontal profile, would reduce the air pressure and, in turn, cut drag. The same would be true for Alex Dowsett's idea of rolling your shoulders in slightly.

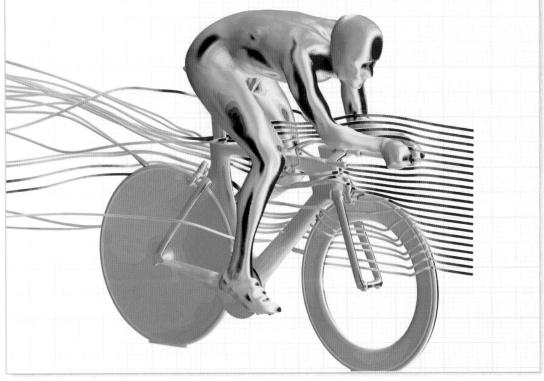

For a good amateur athlete, whose position is streamlined but not as aero as a pro, that'd be more like 0.25–0.30.

This figure becomes even more important when aligned with the power output of a rider. The aim is to generate high wattage and a low CdA – the most efficient combination, as you're not losing power through drag.

When Tony Martin won the 2011 World Time-Trial Championship in Copenhagen, his power output and aerodynamic drag (expressed as watts per square metre CdA) was calculated as 2,089. This compared to 1,943 for Bradley Wiggins in second and 1,725 for Jakob Fulsgang in tenth.

Striking the balance between power output and a low CdA has resulted in a challenge to the old world order, namely, that lower isn't necessarily faster. Look back at footage of French riders, in particular, and they're nearly resting on their top tube. But modern riders position themselves a lot higher.

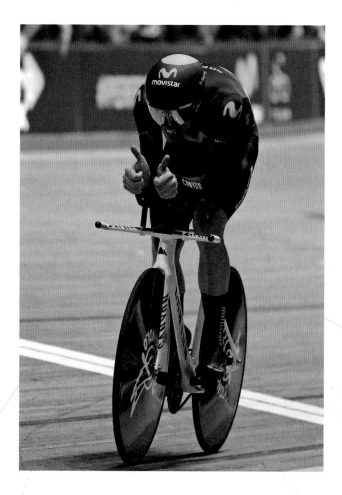

△ Alex Dowsett's blended power and aerodynamics en route to breaking the hour record

## THINNER NOT LOWER

Movistar's Alex Dowsett won Commonwealth time-trial gold for England, broke the hour record as well as blowing the national 10-mile time trial out of the park, his 17 minutes 10 seconds slashing 25 seconds off Michael Hutchinson's time.

'I've spent a lot of time in wind-tunnels and it's affected my position a lot,' says Dowsett. 'I used to be really low but have come up an inch or so since 2009 and that's down to the numbers. If you go too low, it's harder to put down the power. Simon [Smart, aerodynamicist] has brought me up and it's worked, though every so often I have a stupid moment and think I should go a touch further down, but can't generate the power so go back up again!

'Simon also got me to think about the width of my frontal profile and trying to make it more narrow,' Dowsett continues. 'If you watch me in a time trial, I'm constantly bringing my shoulders round and forwards. It helps where your arms and elbows are positioned. If, for instance, you have high edges to the outside of your armrests, that can give you something to push against when you're trying to bring your shoulders in. The sport's moved on but there are still some riders out there who are so low it's ridiculous. They're stuck in the stone ages.'

Why do riders lose power if they're riding lower? When it comes to the aero position, the lower you go, the more the rider compresses the diaphragm, which is the big sheet of muscle at the base of the ribs. The more compressed the diaphragm is, the greater the oxygen cost, tidal volume and breathing frequency. That results in fatigue and lower power output. And that's key, according to Robby Ketchell, data scientist at Team Sky and formerly sports scientist at Garmin-Sharp.

'I remember working with a team in Colorado many years ago and we spent a lot of time putting the riders into super-aerodynamic positions, coming up with numbers that told the rider they only had to produce a reasonable amount of power to go very fast,' says Ketchell. 'The riders said no problem, put me in that position. The problem was, when they went out to the real world and rode at the desired intensity, it just wasn't possible to hold that position and maintain a good power output. So it's always a balance between power output and aerodyamics.'

A multitude of factors influence a rider's sustainable bike position, including their size, flexibility, core strength and lung capacity. Every facet of the object – in this case the rider – has an impact. For instance, wind-tunnel data now suggests that an 'arrow grip' on the bars, with the tips of the fingers touching, gives a 0.54 second saving for every minute ridden at 35mph compared to a rider using a tradi-tional thumbs-inside aerobar grip.

'It all counts,' adds Dowsett, 'though it can be frustrating at times. My gains are becoming more minimal because I've time-trialled for years. So the team are making my teammates faster and they're catching up. Thanks a lot, Simon!'

## TRACK TELEMETRY

The wind-tunnel is a proven weapon in a team's aerodynamic armoury, but teams are conjuring up ever-more technical and cutting-edge methods to give their rider the aerodynamic edge. 'After the Cyclefit bike fit, I headed over to Valencia for track testing,' says Trek-Segafredo's Bauke Mollema.

Now, that might sound an odd strategy for a road team but it's an increasingly useful tactic in the teams' and riders' search toward optimum position. 'Trek take the guys over to Spain, not for racing but to refine their aerodynamics. They hook up the riders and their bikes to various sensors to measure CdA,' says Cavell. It's the next evolutionary step in finding the golden ratio of power output to aerodynamics.

At Specialized, who provide bikes and gear for Astana, Etixx–Quick-Step and Tinkoff Sport, they've created what's grandly termed the Specialized Racing Departmental Program – a department that's directly linked to teams and riders.

 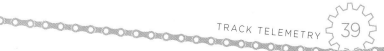

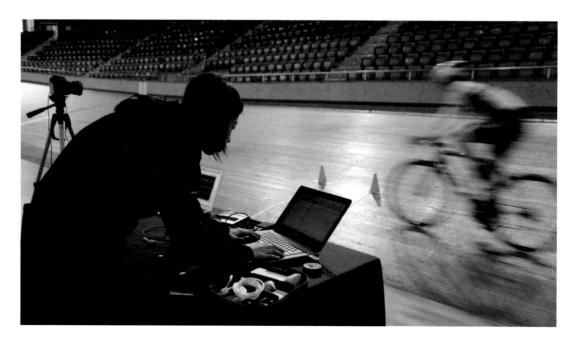

Historically, bike manufacturers supplied Tour teams with bikes for training and racing and that was the deal. Then the sport took off, commercial interest grew and, like their rival bike manufacturers, Specialized now pay sponsorship money as well as supplying bikes, before activating the marketing strategy and waiting for bike sales to rack up.

△ Trek-Segafredo are one of many teams who test their riders' aerodynamics on the track

Now, the relationship has evolved further, as Specialized adopt a more holistic approach by figuring out the best way for riders like Nibali, Kittel and Contador to use their equipment to match the specific goals of the team. The better they do, the more exposure for the brand, and so on.

Chris Yu is aerodynamics Research and Development engineer at Specialized, based in the San Francisco Bay area. He details the lengths the US manufacturer goes to in search of more speed. 'I'll give you an example of how we might work with a GC rider,' he says. 'As soon as the Tour route is announced – usually late October – we begin to get a feel for what the route entails. So if we had a scenario where there's a critical time trial in the middle of the Tour that features a hill in the middle, one of the aims would be: How can we optimise the rider's equipment and power output for that specific TT but still conserve energy for the mountain stages? So we'll put them in our wind tunnel and map them into several different positions, so the rider can play around with them.

'We'll then send them away with those positions before following up with velodrome and on-road testing sessions in Europe later in the season, maybe around late January time,' Yu continues. 'Effectively we retest those positions but

# A battle of physics

○ There are many forces acting on a Tour rider as they battle their way around France. They are:

● **Air resistance:** riders must push air aside to move forward. Above about 14km/h (9mph), it's the most significant force hindering progress. To be precise, air resistance = 0.5 × air density × cycling speed (in still air) squared × the drag coefficient of the rider and bike × the frontal area of the rider and bike.

● **Friction:** this is a force for good and bad. Without it, your tyre wouldn't grip the road and you'd go nowhere. But friction in the drivetrain – essentially the bike's moving parts – can lose about 3 per cent of energy expended.

● **Rolling resistance:** the combined weight of rider and bike misshapes the tyre, losing energy because it doesn't spring back with the same energy that deformed it.

● **Gravity:** this force keeps riders firmly on the ground, but the pull of the earth is also what makes climbing the likes of Alpe d'Huez such a struggle.

▽ Cyclists of the Lotto NL-Jumbo cycling team compete in the first stage of the Giro d'Italia Tour of Italy cycling road race, a 17.6km team time trial race from San Lorenzo al Mare to San Remo, in San Remo on May 9, 2015

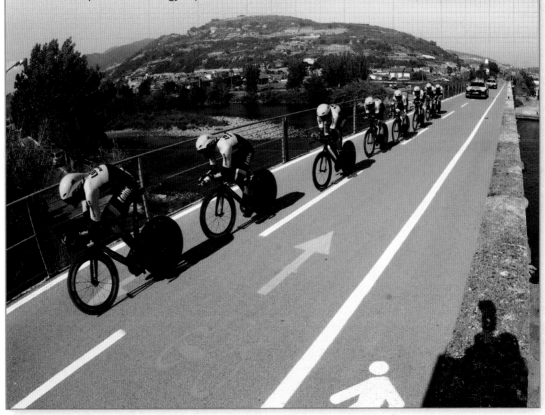

in a slightly different environment where they're racing their bike at race power.

'This is useful but we've now developed telemetry [name given to data collection at one source that's transmitted to receiving equipment] like you'd see in Formula One, which comes down to a number of different sensors. There are the obvious ones like power, drag and speed, but also ones that monitor wind speed and one that tracks the athlete's ride position in real time. We use an infrared laser that monitors torso and head movements while the rider's moving. Another sensor measures lean angle; in other words, how much is he swinging the bike? Both are pretty good indicators of fatigue. The sensors are strapped to the top tube and wirelessly feed information to a trackside server. I can monitor it there or, if I'm in California, I can pick it up here.

'All that data is pushed through software, so we can then paint a more realistic idea of which position will work. We can then tie in that information with information that we have about equipment. We can then run certain power optimisation schemes to calculate which frame, which front wheel, which rear wheel, which tyres, which kit, which helmet and the right position for various sectors to optimise speed and energy expenditure.'

Riders like Alberto Contador now have a menu of positions and gear to choose from depending on the stage. It's impressive stuff and highlights cycling's move toward data and predictive modelling.

▽ Trek-Segafredo testing their riders' aerodynamics on the track

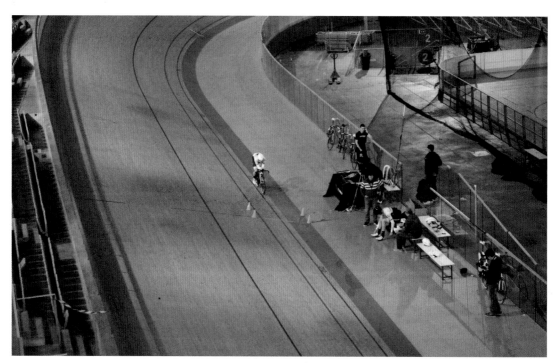

# BEST BIKE SPLIT

TrainingPeaks software recently acquired a company called Best Bike Split. I asked founder Dirk Friel why. 'They've made waves because they've been excellent at correctly predicting the Tour de France time-trial results,' says Friel. 'It's all based on knowing cycling and knowing your algorithms.'

Best Bike Split sucks up a multitude of variables, like power output and the rider's predicted or actual CdA, and can help the rider choose not only pacing strategies but also equipment selection.

The final stage of the 2015 Paris–Nice race is a case in point. It finished with a 9.6km time trial up Col d'Éze just outside Nice. It's short but demanding as it is entirely uphill, its gradient ranging from 3 per cent to 9 per cent. Research has shown that, in general, for the elite riders and their high speeds, aerodynamics is more important than weight. But interestingly that's not quite as clear cut for a stage like Col d'Éze where maintaining an aggressive aero tuck at such steep gradients might result in significantly less power than a road position, due to the lower speeds uphill.

Three Trek Factory Racing riders had undergone velodrome testing earlier in the year, so the support staff had the numbers that mattered including their aerodynamic drag for different bike, wheel and helmet combinations. From this data, Best Bike Split and its algorithms could predict when and where they should come out of the aero tuck and which bike out of the Emoda (road), Speed Concept (time trial) or Emoda with tri-bars would elicit the quickest time. They also included predicted weather conditions on the day based on past meteorological information.

Based on the predictive modelling, Best Bike Split suggested that the Emoda would be the slowest because there were significantly long enough sections that the rider should remain in the aero position. Between the remaining two options, a select band of riders would benefit from the Speed Concept, conserving as much as 15 seconds on the faster sections of the course due to their superior streamlined position and only sacrificing a few seconds on the steeper sections.

But the bike of choice for the majority was the Emoda complete with tri-bars, the lighter weight proving its worth over the steep gradients and the aerobars leading to greater speed over the shallower parts.

'That's what it told Riccardo [Zoidl], who had a good day, finishing just 15 seconds off top 10 in 15th,' says Josu Larrazabel, trainer for Trek-Segafredo. 'Bob Jungels's profile suited both the Speed Concept and the aerobar-fronted Emoda because he's able to produce similar power output on a time-trial bike as a road bike because he's super-flexible. But because of the headwind, it was noted that speed would be less so we again went for the Emoda with aerobars.'

And the result of this impressive piece of information processing? 'Bob had a bad day and finished 49th. Calculations and numbers are very useful but fail to perform at your best and you won't enjoy success at WorldTour level.'

# THE MAN OF DATA

A rider is human after all. Still, data is king and it's something Team Sky has become adept at utilising, so it perhaps came as no surprise when they recruited Robby Ketchell into their ranks at the end of 2014. When Ketchell was at Garmin, he had a broad remit beneath the umbrella of sports science. Sky has given him the more tightly focused role of data scientist, which is a WorldTour first. Issues of confidentiality mean Ketchell is tight-lipped over current projects but he did reveal where he sees the future of racing.

'Predictive analytics is what it's about,' Ketchell enthuses. 'But it's not as easy as just producing a calculation. A lot of times we create this model and, in the real world, it doesn't come anywhere close. So we have to say what we are missing. So you're looking for more data and refinement of interpretation to perfect the model.

'There are variables galore to analyse and cycling is in a really interesting place right now,' he continues. 'There are all these sensors and devices to measure aspects of physiology, movement patterns, biometrics, environment and so on, and doing it in different ways. Key to the future is how you bring that information together. How you aggregate that and bring something meaningful out of it.'

Ultimately, Ketchell's role is to make an unpredictable sport more predictable, and he very much follows Team Sky's ethos of leaving nothing to chance. 'This data-driven approach will reduce the speculative side of racing and tactics,' says Ketchell. 'It's obviously more from the physiology side of things so not the whole picture, though the dream would be reaching a stage where you could measure motivation.'

Ketchell's always been progressive. When Dan Martin jumped clear of the yellow jersey group on the final climb of stage nine at the 2013 Tour de France, it looked like the Irishman's move was based on instinct. In fact, the Garmin-Sharp rider's attack was the result of a perfectly executed set of tactics, planned weeks beforehand and which told Martin how many seconds he'd need at the top of the Hourquette d'Ancizan climb before the descent to Bagnères-de-Bigorre to give himself a chance of victory. That figure was 43 seconds according to Ketchell's calculations and his use of an app he created called Platypus.

Platypus involved real-time data analysis as well as containing information on every rider it was monitoring in that particular stage. 'When riders get into a break, Platypus highlights who the riders are. You can then click on the stats: the breaks they've been in, how often they succeed, and other historical data,' Ketchell said at the time. Directors in the car have access to that information and can make tactical calls based on empirical evidence.

Ketchell says he no longer uses Platypus since moving from Garmin to Team Sky, but working back from specific course challenges and applying training and

> Data is king… key to the future is how you bring that information together.
>
> **Robbie KETCHELL,**
> *Team Sky*

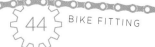

race solutions in advance is becoming a greater goal for every team. That's because mimicking the course you're racing as accurately as possible in training is the ideal when it comes to event preparation. Working on the specific physiological demands of a specific course profile and environmental conditions means the rider can hit the right energy systems for the right duration at the right speed. Psychologically, the rider will also be more confident, knowing exactly what's coming around the next corner or over the next hill.

Of course, Ketchell's not the only data genius swimming around the WorldTour. 'We use an app telling the rider everything they need to know about the race,' says David Bailey, sports scientist at BMC Racing. 'So at Paris–Nice, for instance, they know the schedule, the profile of the course, the weather forecast, what the final 5km looks like and any other useful additional information. For a time trial, it's a lot more detailed.'

Sports scientist David Martin and his team at the Australian Institute for Sport, who worked with Orica GreenEdge and riders of the calibre of Simon Gerrans and Michael Matthews, also left nothing to chance in the build-up to the 2012 London Olympics with what they called 'Project Déjà vu'. 'We recce'd the London course in the build-up and went over with fully instrumented bicycles,' explains Martin. 'They had cameras on, GPS units, accelerometers and power meters. And we videoed the athletes from behind, too. We collected enough information to come back to Australia and program the stationary bicycles with realistic load patterns for the London course. It gave the riders enhanced familiarisation.'

As it transpired, an inspired Bradley Wiggins, fresh from becoming the first Briton to win the Tour de France, took home the men's time-trial gold with sixth-placed Michael Rogers Australia's highest finisher.

'It's certainly a technology we'd use again, though, and there's so many options,' says Martin. 'For instance, in preparation for a hot race, you can put the ergometer [indoor bike] in an environmental bubble so that it replicates a variety of temperatures. So if you knew it was going to be hot, you could crank up the chamber to 30°C and work on different fuelling strategies. If you're in Formula One, this is routine. In cycling this kind of use of technology is starting to come to the fore.'

# REINVENTING THE WHEEL

This progressive approach to cycling is also seen at Specialized's HQ in Morgan Hill, California, where in their own wind tunnel they're refining traditional methods of conserving energy to race faster – drafting – through cutting-edge developments.

'In 2014, unfortunately Mark Cavendish crashed out of the Tour during his mother's stage in Harrogate,' explains Yu, referring to Cavendish's mum who lives in the Yorkshire town. 'It was a shame as we'd introduced new developments into the race build-up. Just before that year's Tour of California, Mark and many of his lead-out train, including Mark Renshaw, visited the wind tunnel.

'The wind tunnel can accommodate more than one rider so we put the riders in, on rollers, and set the wind speed to 65km/h, and ran through different lead-out placements and lay-off distances to see how it affected airflow. A great example of how it can work practically is that Renshaw told us that in many lead-outs, he can feel Cav tapping his rear wheel. That's how close Cav is. So his natural question was: can we have Cav lay off a centimetre or two without losing efficiency and speed?'

Confidentiality means Yu can't divulge the exact results but with the naked eye, Cav still looks pretty close to Renshaw! But it wasn't just how airflow reacted off Renshaw – Specialized took into account the impact that a looming Kittel has on proceedings. 'We measured Cav's efficiency when a large rider like Kittel is behind him, so we borrowed a local cyclist of roughly the size of Marcel and began working out what the effect would be of him sitting on Cav's wheel. We discovered that Cav could actually enjoy a drafting effect from the rider behind.'

That's down to, in this case, Kittel filling the eddy, the swirling of gas when

▽ Mark Cavendish in the best sprinter's green jersey, with Peter Sagan and Edvald Boasson Hagen sprint at the end of the last stage of the 2012 Tour de France to finish at the Champs-Elysees

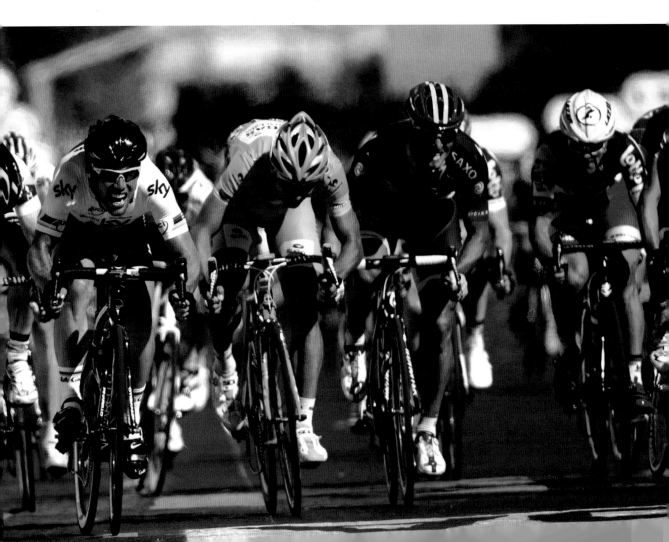

# Drafting: a percentage game

○ Drafting another cyclist is a proven method of conserving energy and, ultimately, pedalling faster and longer. As Professor Bert Blocken and his team at Eindhoven University showed, even the leading cyclist can enjoy an energy saving of 2–3 per cent from the rider behind. Still, those figures are nothing compared to how much the following riders can benefit. And because air pressure increases the faster you ride, the quicker the leading rider, the greater the energy savings for the following rider.

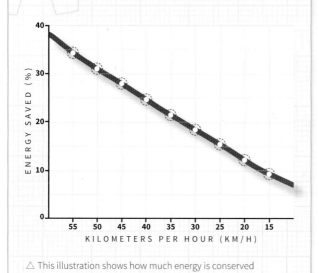

△ This illustration shows how much energy is conserved by the following rider at different speeds.

it passes an object, spinning off Cav's rear wheel, which reduces turbulence. It's a topic that Bert Blocken, professor of physics at Eindhoven University of Technology in the Netherlands, examined in 2012. 'We noticed articles on rally driving that showed if the second car is very close behind the first one, the first one has a lower fuel consumption. So we felt that could work in cycling,' says Blocken.

Blocken and his team sent a team of riders into the wind tunnel and concluded that sitting just 1cm behind gave energy saving benefits of 2–3 per cent for the front rider. At that distance you're bordering on morphing into a tandem but Blocken asserts it's not totally unrealistic. 'While more akin to track riding, on the road cyclists hide behind each other in a staggered fashion, so it's not just one long train linked by just a centimetre. That said, a more real-world 15cm still sees a 1.5 per cent conservation of energy.'

The drafting benefits for the rider behind are more established, of course, and of far greater value. Back in 1979, scientists studied wind resistance and power output in racing groups, measuring a 47 per cent energy saving when following at a rather improbable zero metres, but still a healthy 27 per cent at two metres back. Even at three metres, benefits have been noted.

While it's clearly more energy efficient to sit behind the leading man, teams could use this information to place the rider behind that bit closer to their lead-out man. In turn, the lead-out man could eke out that extra watt or two for that bit longer, which could be the difference between victory and defeat. It's also useful for sports scientists to monitor energy expenditure when it comes to the team time trial and calculating how long each of the nine riders should spend at the front. It's not a lot but remember: this is a world of marginal gains.

# MARGINAL EFFORT

For riders like Felice Gimondi and Barry Hoban who made their names in the 1960s, cycle fit was a more rudimentary affair. One chap held the back wheel up while the rider adopted their 'natural' position. The *directeur sportif* or general manager – there weren't really coaches like there are these days – would then eye up seat height, moving the seat up and down, trying to see if he was 'hitting the spot'. After a few revolutions of the pedal they might drop a plumb line from the knee, the optimum being that it bisected the pedal axle. They'd then fiddle with the stem, changing the length depending on size of rider. They'd write down the physical angles (knee and hip, for instance), note the equipment used and you were done.

When the clock ticked around to the 1980s, technology began to crank up in the world of bike-fitting, partly down to an American outfit called FitKit who created a range of tools that measured dimensions including inseam and quad length that'd theoretically steer you into your optimum position.

Come the late 1990s and early 2000s, as computers and technology evolved, bike-fitting morphed into a whole new world of 3D analysis, real-time feedback and pressure mapping. Outfits like London's Cyclefit have led the way with their intellectual property and equipment squeezing out that extra wattage or two, or cutting one percent of drag from world-class riders like Fabian Cancellara. The days of simply dropping a plumb line from the knee to locate best position are long gone. But whatever your position on the bike, you won't be going anywhere fast if you don't fuel optimally.

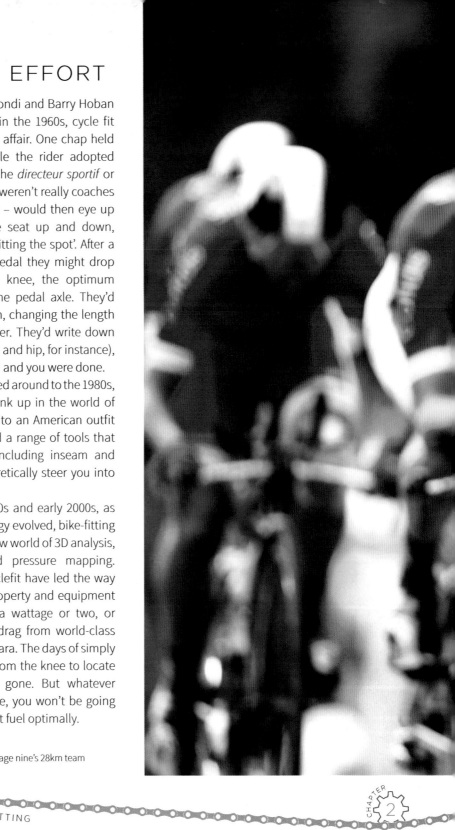

▷ French team Cofidis during stage nine's 28km team time trial at the 2015 Tour

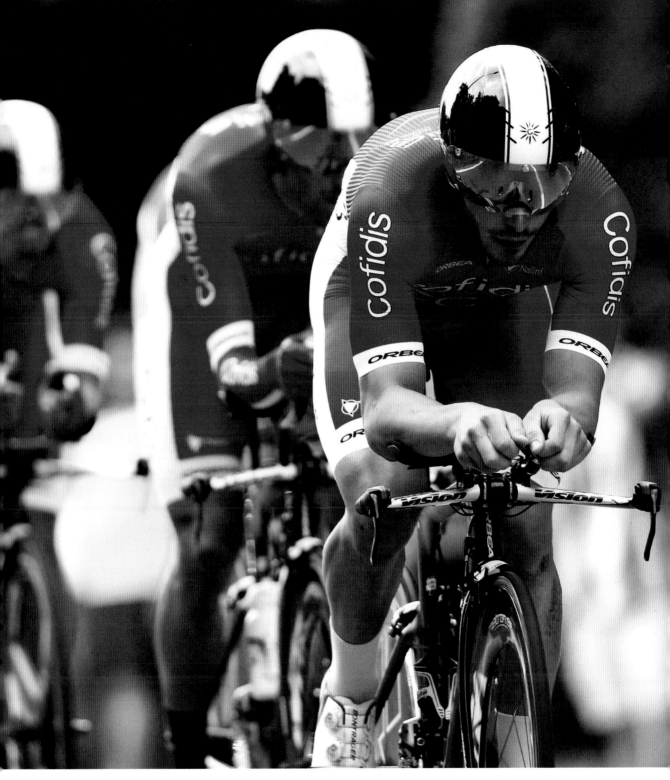

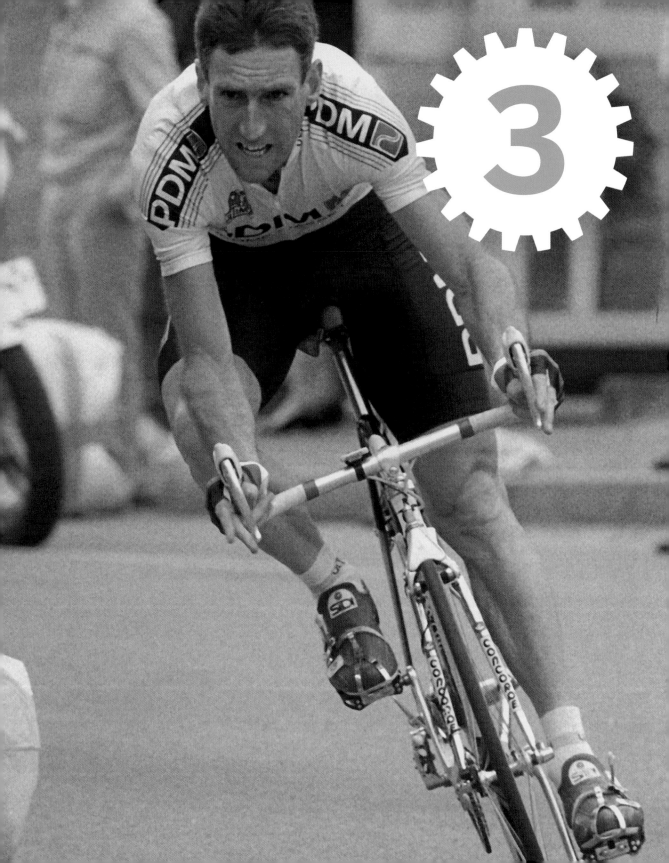

# FUELLING UP TO THE TOUR

'We went to a training camp on the Côte d'Azur. He looked at me and said I'd have to lose weight. I was about twelve-and-a-half stone and perhaps a touch bulky. He told me I had to cut back on food for the next two months – and so began my first taste of de Gribaldy's methods.'

The words of Irish legend Sean Kelly when referring to life under noted *directeur sportif* Jean de Gribaldy, during his first professional race season in 1977 for Flandria. 'We were in a permanent state of hunger,' Kelly continues. 'My meal sizes halved. We'd start with a very small soup and a three-inch nugget of baguette. Main course: chicken, greens and mashed potato. He even removed the doughy part of the bread because he said it took hours to digest. Morning time you'd come down for breakfast and see an oily stain on the tablecloth where De Gribaldy had taken the croissants. But it worked and helped turn me from an out-and-out sprinter to a one-day specialist and GC contender.'

Kelly's racing weight shrunk to just over 11 stone, and victories soon followed, including the first of five career stage wins at the Tour in 1978. He also won Paris–Nice an incredible seven times and Paris–Roubaix twice.

Back in the 1970s and early 1980s, riders would often get by, as Kelly says, on 'chips, gravy and ice-creams, all washed down with a few beers'. Not under de Gribaldy. He was a man ahead of his time and soon became a hated figure to the cyclists under his regime (albeit with grudging respect). de Gribaldy was notable for paying meticulous attention to what a rider put in their body, though based more on instinct and feel than science. Now, professional teams will consult and employ nutritionists, doctors and chefs, trawling the world's universities for the latest research to give their riders a competitive advantage. And when it comes to a rider's general diet, teams are relying increasingly on … fat.

◁ Sean Kelly's obsession with food – or lack of it – was so deep, he penned his autobiography 'Hunger'

# FAT FOUNDATION

▽ Good fats form a core part of a rider's off-season diet, including at training camps

'You see it with the Sky riders, they show up in February and they are incredibly lean. That's because they've been on a ketogenic [high fat] diet through the winter months and encouraged the body to burn fat, which tends to pare down your total mass by quite a bit. It's quite a change from my racing days when it all used to be about the carbohydrates.' So reveals the charismatic Jonathan Vaughters, former professional rider and current manager of Cannondale-Garmin.

While carbohydrates still rule when it comes to racing the Tour, recent times have seen a shift in the composition of a professional rider's general diet. Where once fat was demonised, now it's a mainstay of the WorldTour larder.

'Some of our riders' diets can comprise up to 35 per cent in fats and it's at the upper end of that during the off-season,' says BMC Racing's nutritionist Judith Haudum. 'Of course, the emphasis here is on polyunsaturated and monosaturated fatty acids, so the intake of saturated fats is low. Beyond lean meats and fish, we include a variety of plant-based foods because they contain healthy fats. I'm talking olives, olive oil, flax, nuts and avocado.'

'The good fats are vital,' adds Haudum, 'though more important before race season.' It's a salient point as macronutrient composition is affected by exercise intensity. Research suggests that when training at 50 per cent of maximal aerobic capacity, 45–55 per cent of calories used derive from fat. This drops to about 10–30 per cent when training at 75 per cent of maximum and zero when you are flat out and ascending Alpe d'Huez. So, broadly speaking, the riders' diets should reflect this change in intensity. And as the general intensity of riding remains slightly lower during the off-season, the riders will be generating proportionally greater energy from fat than carbohydrates. Carbohydrates become more important during race season.

So in pre-season Tinkoff Sport team chef Hannah Grant focuses on recipes that are swimming in fatty

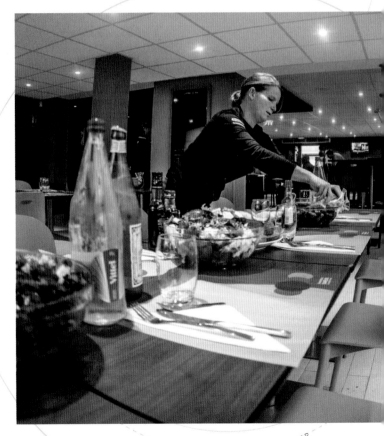

goodness and, more importantly, taste. 'One of the cooked salmon dishes the riders go particularly crazy for is salmon baked with ginger, honey and orange. In that dish you also enjoy the benefits of the anti-inflammatory ginger,' says Grant. 'Sushi is always a winner, and the Danish classic gravlax – which consists of fennel, dill and pepper-cured salmon with sweet mustard sauce and vegetable crudités – is also high on the list of favourites.' (For more information on race nutrition see Chapter 9.)

Beyond the taste, fat is so calorie dense that, with a healthy supply of oxygen, it can generate huge amounts of energy. Physiologist Allen Lim, who has worked with a number of professional teams including BMC Racing and Garmin-Sharp, says that an average Tour rider weighs 154lb (70kg). At 3,500 calories per pound of fat, a rider weighing 150lbs with just 8 per cent body fat has 12lbs of stored fat, which is the equivalent of 42,000 calories. It's why even the most sinewy cyclist can spend much of a stage burning fat without detriment to their performance or health.

The nutritionist and chef will also ensure omega-3 forms a key part of the diet. Mountains of research show that omega-3 protects the heart, controls blood pressure and maintains a lean body weight. Omega-3 also benefits blood and muscle functions by acting as a cleanser, making blood less sticky and more fluid.

'This allows more oxygen to reach the cyclist's brain and muscles, ensuring faster riders,' explains Grant. 'Cold-pressed flax-seed oil is high in omega-3, which is why I add it to the riders' smoothies in the morning. We make sure many of the meals we cook contain foods high in omega-3 like chia seeds, salmon, nuts and mackerel.'

Omega-3 also displays cannibalistic tendencies: it consumes fat. According to researchers at Washington University School of Medicine in St Louis, omega-3 helps break down existing fat by activating fat-burning pathways through the liver. But omega-3's most important properties are anti-inflammatory, reducing inflammation racked up from thousands of miles of riding and boosting the immune system.

British Cycling's use of fish oils is legendary – under Nigel Mitchell, who then moved to Team Sky, the riders took two grams of high-quality fish oil a day. The oil contains a fatty acid (eicosapentaenoic acid) that reduces muscle breakdown when the muscles are stressed through exercise and improves protein synthesis. It was something Mitchell brought in from the NHS, when he was working in cancer care; he used it to help patients keep muscle tone. Just to highlight the importance Team Sky attribute to good fats, they also have their own brand of extra-virgin olive oil purely for the team.

Another benefit of fat is that testosterone, which has received such a bad press through the actions of numerous nefarious riders, is made up from cholesterol. Naturally produced testosterone is a good thing as it's involved in many performance-enhancing processes, like building muscle. Lower testosterone levels are one of the clearest signs of overtraining, so a diet higher in good fats will stabilise testosterone structures, increase their levels and send the rider back to full health. The rider's body converts the cholesterol in fat to steroidal hormones, of which testosterone is one.

Unlike carbohydrates, a diet high in fats has been proven to satiate appetite, which is why many teams employ this higher-fat option during the off-season. If you feel fuller you'll find it easier to keep your weight at an optimum. With no races on the calendar and recovering from the mental fatigue of the previous year's competition, it's a common occurrence for riders to pile on a few early-off-season pounds. 'I'm one of the fortunate ones as I might only put on 2–3kg at most,' says Lotto-Soudal's Greg Henderson. 'I know some riders who could easily put on 8–9kg.' Clearly, in a sport where weight significantly dictates outcome, playing catch-up from the season's start isn't a desirable position.

## Energy production

○ Fat is the muscles' primary fuel for low- to moderate-intensity exercise. Carbohydrate is the muscles' primary fuel for moderately high to high-intensity exercise and is stored in a form known as glycogen (in plants it's called starch).

Glycogen stores are limited in the muscles and liver – the primary storage spots in the body – coming in at around 500g for well-trained cyclists. As a gram of carbohydrate contains four calories, that's around 2,000 calories of energy, and is why recreational runners, for example, will 'hit the wall' in a marathon at around 21 miles. They've been running at an intensity that's simply left their glycogen bank empty three hours in. However, because fat stores are plentiful, if a rider can increase their reliance on fat fuel and decrease carbohydrate reliance during relatively intense riding, in theory the professional peloton could delay fatigue and cycle stronger.

South African researchers examined the effects of a high-fat diet versus a normal diet (in both cases prior to carbohydrate loading) on fuel metabolism and cycling time-trial performance. Five trained cyclists undertook two 14-day trials where they consumed either a 65 per cent fat diet or their habitual 30 per cent fat diet for 10 days, before switching to a 70 per cent carbohydrate diet for three days.

All subjects then performed a cycling test consisting of two and a half hours at 70 per cent of peak oxygen uptake followed by a 20km time trial. The high-fat diet resulted in increased total fat oxidation and reduced total carbohydrate oxidation during exercise. More importantly, the high-fat treatment led to improved time-trial times. On average, the cyclists completed the 20km time trial 4.5 per cent faster after the high-fat diet. Protein can also be burnt to release energy (like carbohydrate, 1g of protein = 4kcals). However, this is unfavourable as it breaks down muscle.

# THE FATMAX ZONE

There's also evidence that consuming more good fats – rather than manmade fats that, among a myriad of badness, clog arteries and raise cholesterol – and with targeted training, increases something called your 'Fatmax', the intensity at which you're burning the most fat for fuel. This concept emanated from noted exercise physiologist Dr Asker Jeukendrup of Birmingham University, UK, who, via a series of gas analysis measurements, calculated the proportion of energy derived from carbohydrates and fat as exercise intensity increased. The Fatmax test lasts about 20 to 45 minutes depending on the rider's fitness. The test starts at a low intensity of power but increases every 3 minutes with carbon dioxide and oxygen levels monitored.

From the research, Jeukendrup observed that the 'best' Fatmax zone was around 60–63 per cent $VO_2$ max, or around 75 per cent of maximum heart rate. For less fit individuals, this dropped to 50 per cent $VO_2$ max. Why is this important?

'Carbohydrate is the gasoline and fat is the diesel,' says Movistar sports scientist Mikel Zabala. 'There's evidence that the higher a rider's Fatmax is, the more they can reserve glycogen levels for important parts of the race. And that's why many riders often train in a glycogen-depleted state.'

The science behind how energy production fluctuates depending on exercise intensity is detailed further in the 'Energy production' box opposite, but it's clear that this low-carbohydrate template is becoming more popular throughout the professional peloton. According to research, it transforms the body into a fat-burning machine and so, ultimately, spares glycogen for high-intensity moments like all-out sprints or kicking on a hill.

Dr James Morton of John Moores University, UK, and nutritionist at Team Sky, explains the physiology behind the thinking: 'The main adaptation your body makes when you do a glycogen-depleted or water-only training session is enhanced mitochondrial volume in your muscles. That means all the enzymes and sites of aerobic metabolism are more active.'

The phenomenon is known as mitochondrial biogenesis, and as a result of these changes, you become more efficient at using fat for fuel at a given exercise intensity, which means you produce less lactate – and less fatiguing hydrogen ions – so conserve glycogen.

Intensity is key here. Once you tip over your Fatmax, your body burns an ever-increasing amount of carbohydrates, which is why low-carbohydrate diets go hand-in-hand with low- to moderate-intensity sessions.

That's the theory, but what do the riders think of these glycogen-depleted sessions? 'I find them useful for preparing my body to perform at the end of a race,' says Koen de Kort, a key member in Giant-Alpecin's lead-out train, 'although we primarily do them in the off-season when building up to races.'

There are many models of training 'fasted'. Historically the most common involved the rider awaking fasted, before knocking back a water and espresso and heading out the door. That's not how it works at Giant. 'For breakfast we might have only high-fat foods – maybe an avocado or some nuts,' de Kort explains. 'We'll then go for a relatively easy three-hour ride. After the ride we'll refuel but again with no carbohydrates – just protein and fat. We'll then go for another ride, this time cycling for around 2.5 hours. Again, it'll be low effort with some medium-intensity intervals thrown in. After that last effort, we'll refuel on carbohydrates.'

It's all designed to supercharge de Kort's body to metabolise fat instead of carbohydrates at a higher-intensity of cycling and the 32-year-old appreciates its benefits on performance, if not his state of being. 'You do feel more lethargic and it all feels a little like you are training in slow motion; in fact, you do cycle slower but, ultimately, you'll be faster come the races.'

## NEW 'TRAIN FASTED' THEORIES

That feeling of lethargy and near-illness is something John Hawley, Professor and head of the Exercise and Nutrition Research Group at Australian Catholic University, has recently co-authored a study about – focusing on the new concept of 'sleeping extremely low', which builds on the work of University of Copenhagen physiologists who devised the original 'train low, race high' protocol back in 2005. They mooted the idea that riders could perform a glycogen-depleted session every second day by eating a normal breakfast (porridge) to fuel their morning sessions but then skipping lunch to leave the muscles depleted of glycogen come the second session. The problem is, that method of training had a negative impact on the rider's state of being.

'No one wants to feel rubbish and like their power output is plummeting, especially professional cyclists,' says Hawley. 'In fact, we showed that training with low glycogen reduces power output by around 7–8 per cent. That's the difference between 1st and 451st! So we ran a trial where the riders took no carbs but caffeine instead, which stimulates the fat metabolism and lowers perception of effort, and that rescued things to 3.5 per cent.'

But still athletes 'felt terrible'. 'That's when we thought it was time to get smart,' says Hawley. 'We did not want to compromise their training intensity but we did want them to train "low" some of the time. So we had guys come into the laboratory last thing at night. They performed a high-intensity session and then went to bed fasted. So train low, sleep with low glycogen stores, which is ultimate periodisation. You wake up fasted, have no breakfast and everything to do with fat metabolism is elevated. Then you do your lower-intensity exercise but it isn't compromised. You get the best of both worlds. You train high in the evening, sleep low – and, more importantly, none of the subjects slept badly.'

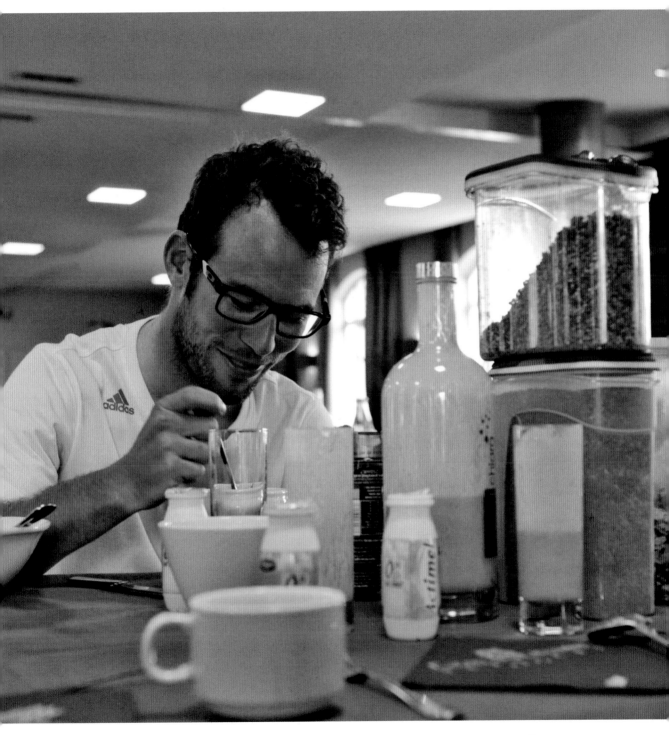

It's an evolving field with innovators like Hawley stretching the physiological knowledge base. But it is one thing working in the lab – it is another trying out a potentially energy-depleting protocol on riders whose careers rely on results.

'There's irrefutable evidence that if you do low-glycogen training in a certain way, you'll enjoy a benefit,' says Tinkoff Sport's former head of sports science Daniel Healey. 'Essentially it's fitness gains for free. The problem is we've had riders on the team who, in the past, have had a negative experience with it. I'm not going to start gambling with one of the best teams in the world on something that's still quite experimental. We're still looking for gains in more proven ways.'

Still, research and real-life application of tapping into fat reserves is an area of increased focus and will no doubt evolve over the next few seasons. And don't be surprised if Team Sky lead the way. 'I know that there's talk that Sky has been using ketone drinks to spare glycogen for the tough, important sections of a race,' says Henderson, who raced for Team Sky between 2010 and 2011, and claimed victory in Sky's first-ever race, the Cancer Council Helpline Classic, back in 2010.

Team Sky hasn't commented on their ketone usage but, according to David Holdsworth of Oxford University, who leads current research into ketone-based drinks, when talking to British magazine *Cycling Weekly*, 'There are professional teams and world-famous cyclists who've used ketones for significant events, which they've won.'

These drinks are said to cost as much as £2,000 per litre so would require a team with deep pockets. They're designed to spare glycogen reserves with studies showing a small increase in the time it takes to ride to exhaustion; in other words, you can rider harder for longer. That and fat utilisation for performance is certainly an area that's been looked into by Jonathan Vaughters, team manager at Cannondale-Garmin, but, he says, there are caveats.

'You can overdo that and start burning muscle tissue so it's something that has to be monitored closely,' he explains. 'Get it right, go to the race after normalising your carbohydrate content and your body should tap into fat stores better. That's a big change from 10 years ago when I was racing. Then it was all about carbohydrates all-year round. Mind you, carbs are still vital when you're racing and the intensity is higher.'

# PERIODISATION OF NUTRITION

That's where the concept of periodised nutrition comes in and is where the fuel you consume matches the needs of your training. It begins with higher fats in the off-season but, as the race season picks up, there's a greater focus on carbohydrate intake to fuel the higher-intensity riding.

That increase in carbohydrates derives from three key areas: general meals (including more pasta and rice), an increase in carbohydrate snacking including fruit and a greater use of sports foods. Healthy snacking keeps the riders' glycogen levels topped up to maximise training efficiency, especially as training twice a day is a common occurrence. In fact, their importance to the Tour riders in order to maintain the intensity and duration of sessions required for a three-week stage races shouldn't be underestimated.

'I know they're important for racing and high-intensity training but I'm not a huge fan of carbs,' says Team Sky's Nicolas Roche. But it turns out that carbs suit him best: 'In the past I've tried a high-fat diet but, sadly, it didn't work out. Now I'm back to pasta when racing. Ultimately, everyone has a different metabolism. Someone whose is high might be able to eat more fat, or more oily stuff, than someone who has a slow metabolism.'

Periodisation of nutrition not only serves the specific physiological demands of training, it can also increase or decrease a rider's weight depending on the goal event. While Vaughters says that someone like Dan Martin typically maintains a stable weight throughout the year, the German rider Jan Ullrich was renowned for beefing up during the off-season. He countered criticism of his weight gain with the pithy reply, 'I have seen many lean riders in the peloton, but very few Tour winners'. Ullrich's reply clearly has holes: there's not a huge amount of fat on Nibali.

Team Dimension Data's performance biochemist Rob Child is a proponent of periodisation of nutrition. He's used it in the past to great success with Thor Hushovd and it's something he has carried over to the African team. 'We use periodisation to manage goal races and race weight,' says Child. 'Let's take Steve Cummings. Looking back at the start of 2015, his nutrition strategy worked well: his power-to-weight ratio was good and he was recovering well after sessions. But we needed to reduce his weight from the classics for the Tour de France, so after Liège we began working on reducing body fat, and perhaps a degree of muscle mass, so he would drop to around 70–71kg come the Utrecht prologue. Like it did for Thor, it'll help him on the climbs.'

Why the difference in weight between classics and the Tour de France? Child argues that race weight should be higher in the tough, cobbled classics, not only to conquer the punchy climbs and stretches of cobbles, but also to fight the chances of infection. 'For whatever reason, there is less chance of picking up an infection in the summer, when we might want Steve to drop from, say, 8.5 per cent body fat to 6 per cent. That philosophy is not for all, though. Look at the French. They like to see their guys super-lean all the time. To me, that simply raises the chances of catching an illness.'

While a high-fat diet helps to reduce a rider's weight during the winter, protein performs a similar role during the race season, when the intensity of sessions is higher. Protein not only repairs the body and so reduces the chances of over-

> ❝ I've tried a high-fat diet but it didn't work out. Now I'm back to pasta when racing. ❞
>
> Nicolas ROCHE, *Team Sky*

training, it satiates appetite. Team Sky often fuel longer rides with energy bars with high-protein content and, like glycogen-depleted training, it's an area of growing focus for WorldTour teams.

'We used to think protein was really just for muscle heads,' says nutrition and exercise expert Hawley. 'I had a bodybuilding mate who worked down the corridor from me and he used to stink of tuna. That's because he had been eating protein right throughout the day. He was right to because it's good for muscle repair, but it's also vital for endurance athletes.'

In the journal *Applied Physiology, Nutrition and Metabolism*, in a 2014 article entitled 'Beyond muscle hypertrophy: why dietary protein is important for endurance athletes', Hawley and his team looked at the role protein plays in enhancing performance in endurance athletes. The researchers observed that after aerobic efforts, the body sends a stress signal that directs amino acids to build so-called mitochondrial proteins; in the case of weight training, it directs the amino acids toward creating contractile proteins, which help to construct muscle fibres.

Mitochondria are the powerhouse of muscles, and it's the biological kitchen in which carbohydrate and fat is burned for fuel, so by increasing protein content, you're increasing your efficiency at using carbohydrate and fat. More protein, better performing mitochondria, resulting in a more efficient 'boiler' essentially – key for high performance endurance athletes.

'In our study, we suggest that the endurance athlete should ingest a 20g dose of protein straight after the ride,' says Hawley. 'Endurance athletes should aim for around one gram per kilogram body weight of protein – though that should be more

## Protein-packed diet

○ BMC's nutritionist Judith Haudum serves up a training-day protein-based menu for rides of around three to four hours. This would be for riders like Rohan Dennis and Greg van Avermaet.

● **Breakfast (2-3 hours before ride):** Porridge with nuts and dried fruits, wholegrain bread with butter and jam, small low-fat yoghurt, fruit, coffee with milk.
● **During the ride:** One PowerBar Energize bar, five apricots or dried figs, one banana, one bottle of sports drink, two bottles of water.
● **Post-ride:** Milk-fruit-smoothie containing 500ml milk, one banana and two tablespoons

of honey. Or bowl of cereal with milk or yoghurt and one tablespoon of honey. Or 30g protein (whey) with milk and honey or jam sandwich.
● **Lunch:** Roasted chicken breast, wholegrain pasta, mixed salad; fruit salad.
● **Snacks:** Small bowl of cereal, fruit, granola bar.
● **Dinner:** Vegetable soup, steak fillet with potatoes and vegetables, piece of cake.

for professional cyclists – and consumed at regular intervals throughout the day.'

'I'd make sure riders are getting at least two grams protein per kilogram body weight,' adds Healey. 'I'd suggest that there's an argument that protein requirements are even greater for endurance athletes than bodybuilders.' Hawley suggests front-loading protein – in other words, making sure you have a dosage or two before lunch – maximises gains from morning training sessions.

As for the type of protein Philippe Gilbert and co. will be ingesting over at BMC Racing, here is the team's nutritionist Judith Haudum: 'If we want the protein to enter the riders' systems quickly, we will go for whey because it is readily absorbed. Hence, it is useful for recovery after long training rides. Casein protein is absorbed more slowly, so is good during not only the day but also at night.'

# ANTIOXIDANT IMPORTANCE

It's not all about the macronutrients fat, carbohydrate and protein, of course, as highlighted by the Paris Cardiovascular Centre in a study that showed Tour riders lived an average 6.3 years longer than the general public. Their stronger hearts and lungs certainly helped, as did a diet that fought illness and infection. What is the magic ingredient?

'This is where antioxidants come in,' says Healey. Attend the team's training camp and the buffet before your eyes resembles a rainbow. Reds and oranges, yellows and green, it is a colourful optical feast. A diet rich in fruit and vegetables is an excellent source of antioxidants and ensures the riders recover more efficiently for the next session.

Healey's performance archive features a food sheet that explains to the riders the importance of the ORAC (oxygen radical absorption capacity) scale. This grandiose title measures the antioxidant capacity of foods, so the higher the score, the bigger the benefit. A snapshot of foods high in antioxidants include: plums (7,581 on the ORAC scale), pecan nuts (17,947), broccoli (2,386), cranberry (9,584) and Jonathan Vaughters's favourite, red wine (5,043).

'All you have to do to supercharge your health during periods of hard training or after a race is include foods with the highest ORAC score in your daily intake as often as you can,' says Healey. 'It is that simple.'

According to Child, antioxidants are of particular importance during the winter months when the chances of picking up an infection are at their greatest. 'There are lots of reasons why you might become ill during the winter, including reduced levels of vitamin D from the sun,' he says. 'Also, if you're training in colder and wetter climes, you will be riding on dirty roads. If you're in the UK, say, and cruise past a farm, they could have been spraying the field with liquidised cowpat. That means each time you take a swig from your bottle, you're ingesting a fair load of bacteria.'

Everyone naturally eats more fruit and vegetables when it is hot, so it's an area teams diligently encourage their riders to focus on during the off-season – by any means. When Nigel Mitchell was nutritionist on Team Sky, he ensured riders had at least a litre of juice each day – a juice with every meal. Carrots, ginger and celery became staples with pineapple juice reducing viscosity to make it more drinkable.

Mitchell also juiced mountains of beetroot. Beetroot juice and their performance enhancing properties have received a great deal of press these past few years. The idea is that, when digested, nitrates within the beetroot flow into a biochemical pathway in the body that converts them to nitric oxide. Studies have shown this conversion has the effect of reducing the oxygen cost of low-intensity exercise and extending time to exhaustion during high-intensity exercise.

Professor Andy Jones is the man behind the beetroot phenomenon. One of his more recent experiments into beetroot, in 2013, saw him and his team at Exeter University take 10 healthy males and have them consume one, two or four shots of a concentrated form of beetroot called 'Beet It' two and a half hours before moderate to high-intensity cycling. They found that taking two or four shots of beetroot juice reduced $VO_2$ levels during moderate-intensity exercise – in other words, exercise felt easier – with two shots performing better than four, lengthening efforts by 14 per cent and 12 per cent, respectively.

'Some of the guys go for chronic supplementation so as part of their salad, they'll always have beetroot in it,' says Dr Jonathan Baker, sports scientist at Team Dimension Data. 'Some will have a vegetable smoothie in the morning with beetroot, celery, carrots, lime… and have it every day so they're always topping up. It becomes part of their routine. And some of our riders will have Beet It.'

Companies like Beet It take all these beetroots and essentially juice them into a more concentrated form. So you can buy a litre bottle of essentially juiced beetroot. 'It's pretty unpleasant but, within three or four days, you do notice a difference in oxygen efficiency,' says Baker, though the Englishman isn't totally convinced of its merits. 'We have done tests in the lab via looking at work rate and oxygen uptake and compared with past results, and you might see half a percent of difference, if that. And is it really from the beetroot juice? You don't know. Many use it anyway as it doesn't do any harm.'

'We tried beetroot but the results were questionable,' adds Teun van Erp, sports scientist at Giant-Alpecin. 'We didn't notice significant performance benefits and many of the riders were put off by the taste.'

This ambivalence in the elite ranks is supported by research from Wilkerson in 2012, who showed that performance effects were less evident in elite athletes, partly because their metabolism and oxygen transfer is already so efficient. 'Beetroot is a relatively new trend but I'm not convinced,' says Marcel Kittel, the Etixx–Quick-Step sprinter.

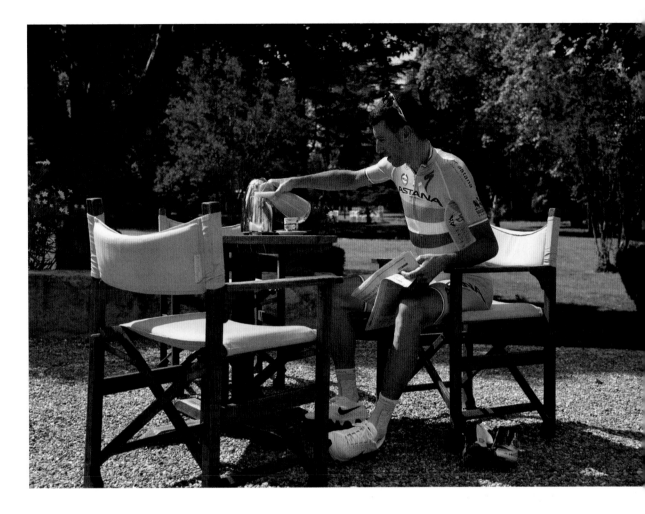

△ Italy's Vincenzo
Nibali, the overall
leader's yellow jersey,
pours himself a glass
of orange juice during
a rest day as part
of the 2014 Tour
de France

# GLUTEN-FREE DIET

Another nutritional tactic 'enjoyed' by riders is adhering to a gluten-free diet. At first that might sound abhorrent to a professional who has been raised on pasta and bread, but is something the Garmin-Transitions team famously followed in the build-up and during the 2010 Tour de France.

The reasons behind the decision were that Dr Allen Lim, former exercise physiologist, and Vaughters, thought that by removing gluten – a composite of proteins in wheat – it would make the riders' bodies more efficient at processing carbohydrates and not become bloated or distressed . They also knew that the team could get enough carbohydrates from other means.

'I was pleasantly surprised,' said team leader Christian Vande Velde at the time, who, very much leading from the front, was the first member of the team to experiment with going wheat-free. 'I just had all-around better digestion, and digestion is the biggest thing in utilising the energy I consume.' Teammate Tom Danielson had a similar experience when he started following the diet during the Tour of Missouri in 2008, citing improved digestion, better sleep and faster recovery as three major benefits.

The theory is that humans are ill-equipped to digest wheat. Unlike cows, humans lack the enzymes in our saliva and stomach to fully breakdown and absorb gluten for nutritional use. It's an issue Lotto-Soudal's Greg Henderson wrestled with 10 years ago before being diagnosed as gluten-intolerant.

'I had numerous stops in cornfields and the side roads because of a bad stomach,' explains Henderson. 'Now I can easily manage it by replacing pasta with potatoes, for instance. Mind you, going out for dinner is still a dangerous place. You might have a lovely night out with the wife, then come the next morning you're feeling pretty rough. I'm lying there thinking I'm sure I only had some meat and potatoes, how am I feeling so crook? But then you remember the meat had a sauce, which must have contained flour.'

Henderson also reveals that his race nutrition is oat-free (oats are gluten-free but many oats are processed in facilities with wheat and so could be contaminated) with 'particularly good choices coming out of America'. The New Zealander has clearly managed the situation well, with many stage victories to his name including the Vuelta and Paris–Nice.

Henderson also discloses that he takes a branched-chain amino-acid supplement called Sanas before bed to boost recovery from training. In the past, he has also experimented with medium-chain triglycerides. 'They didn't particularly work for me but there is some interesting science behind them,' he says.

> ❝ There are vegetarians on our team… but it requires more planning to keep the diet balanced and consume all the essential nutrients. ❞
>
> **Judith HAUDUM,** *BMC Racing*

Before Dr Asker Jeukendrup and his team discovered that riders could absorb more than 60g of carbohydrates when training through a combination of glucose and fructose (see Chapter 9 on race nutrition for more information) they investigated whether medium-chain triglycerides could act as an additional fuel source. MCTs are fats but relatively small fats, meaning they can break down and be absorbed into the body quickly.

In the first of a series of studies, the good doctor added MCTs to a carbohydrate drink and the results showed that, yes, MCTs oxidised rapidly and completely. But because the team only gave relatively small amounts of MCT – just 30g over the course of 3 hours – no changes were seen in metabolism or performance. 'Just dish up more MCT,' you might think. The problem is, any more and riders began to experience abdominal problems. And those who could manage greater MCT

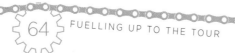

intake actually saw a decrease in sprint performance. In short, if Henderson had continued to ride the MCT path, he could have ended up unemployed.

As well as going gluten-free, Garmin attracted nutritional headlines when one of their riders, American Dave Zabriskie, became the first documented vegan to race the Tour de France. So no meat, dairy or cheese, though he cheated slightly by eating small amounts of salmon twice a week to increase iron absorption. It started well, with Zabriskie helping Garmin win the team time trial and get Thor Hushovd into yellow. That's where Hushovd remained until stage nine, which turned out to be the end of the American's race after badly injuring his wrist in a crash. Still, Zabriskie showed it is possible to perform at the highest level without meat.

'There are vegetarians on our team, too,' says Haudum of her BMC Racing charges, though concedes it's practically more challenging. 'Because many plant-based protein sources don't contain all the amino acids, it requires some more planning to keep the diet balanced and consume all the essential nutrients, especially at races and during intense phases.

'And there is, of course, the challenge with iron. Red meat is a good source and without consuming meat, one needs to make sure the other iron sources are included into the diet, like kale and brown rice. Foods that are included to cover protein needs depend on the type of vegetarian you are. If you eat dairy and eggs, then foods would be dairy products and eggs, fish, soy and soy-based products (tofu), legumes and nuts.'

On the plus side for vegetarian athletes, it means the nutritionists don't have to concern themselves with clenbuterol, the illegal performance enhancer that led to the UCI stripping Alberto Contador of his 2010 Tour de France title despite the Spanish rider claiming it came from contaminated meat. The Court of Arbitration for Sport (CAS) actually partly agreed. It ruled his positive was 'likely [due to a] contaminated food supplement than by a blood transfusion or the ingestion of contaminated meat' but still banned him for two years and stripped his Tour title. (Clenbuterol is often used in cattle farming to relax the uterus in cows when giving birth, and that's how it ends up in the food chain.)

'Problems can stem from not looking into the exact origin of the meat that might be served at a training camp or race,' says Etixx–Quick-Step nutritionist Peter Hespel. 'Of course, as professionals we're all more diligent now and make sure we do so, especially as some countries' legislation into hormone use in cattle isn't that strict. Given the fact that current doping detection techniques can find trace amounts of hormone, even a biologically insignificant hormone can result in a positive doping test.'

Professional cyclists' diets in the modern era are more strictly controlled than in times gone by thanks to nutritionists and chefs setting out nutritional programmes at training camps and encouraging riders to follow them when they're cycling at home. Though Trek-Segafredo's head chef Kim Rokkjaer says you still

 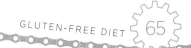

# Fuelled by vitamins

○ Vitamins are essential for maximising performance. The Tour de France arguably stresses the human mind and body like no other sporting event. For 21 stages, the riders must consume enough calories to fuel peak performance. But they must also ensure their vitamin levels are sufficient to keep their metabolism running smoothly and to avoid infection. Here are four key vitamins that keep the riders rolling toward Paris.

● **Vitamin C:** Vitamin C is projected as the first defence against colds and upper respiratory tract infections – common when overexerting yourself – but research is equivocal on whether heavy doses kill colds any faster than the recommended daily amount of around 90mg. Where it's of more use is keeping capillary walls and blood vessels firm for better blood flow – useful when riding at high intensity. 'It also improves iron absorption, which has clear cycling benefits as iron helps oxygen bind to blood that's then delivered to working muscles,' says nutritionist Lucy-Ann Prideaux. There's an argument that you shouldn't take vitamin C straight after training as research shows it could blunt the adaptation process but this shouldn't be too much of an issue at the Tour. Just half a red pepper or one large orange will cover the daily allowance.

● **Vitamin D:** There's evidence that good levels of vitamin D (around 95–124mmol/l) reduce inflammation and thereby the time riders will feel stiff and sore post-ride. Vitamin D can be found in egg yolks, fatty fish such as wild salmon and trout, and fortified milk and cereals – but only about 10 per cent of the amount you need. Uniquely, the rest is through sunlight, which is clearly not an issue come the French summer. 'That's why many believe reductions in vitamin D levels explains the increase in winter coughs, colds and even influenza,' says Dr Will Mangar, head of blood-profiling outfit InDurance.

● **Vitamin B1 (thiamin):** B1 could be deemed the cyclist's most vital vitamin as it plays a pivotal role in converting glucose into energy (as do vitamins B6 and B12), which comes in handy when the riders are projecting along above their Fatmax zone (see page 55). B1 also strengthens the nervous system for more efficient pedalling. Around 1.4mg of B1 daily is recommended to keep healthy. This is the equivalent of a cup of unsalted peanuts, three cups of lentils or four servings of asparagus. But as vitamin B1 is prone to heat destruction through cooking, a supplement might be needed.

● **Vitamin E:** The antioxidant vitamin E helps to sweep up free radicals that are the by-product of metabolism, so it's key to strengthening the immune system. Like vitamin C, though, there's evidence that significant amounts can hamper cellular adaptations in the working muscles. Recommended daily allowance is 4mg, which is easily ticked off with around 150g of almonds or a healthy serving of spinach. As vitamin E is stored in the fat, and not lost in urine, a supplement is not usually necessary.

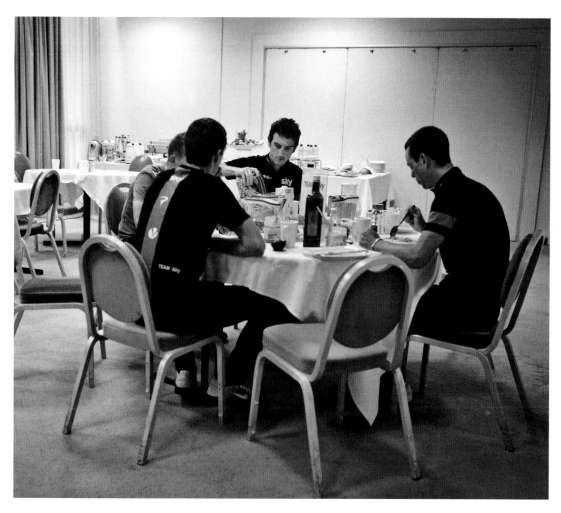

▽ Team Sky with the obligatory bottle of olive oil in the foreground

can't monitor them all the time. 'But they're professional,' he adds. 'They won't want to gorge and pile on the pounds. They know it'd just slow them down.'

Food and cycling have forever ridden hand in hand, though most have been aware that the lighter you are, the quicker you'll ride. Bernard Hinault, for instance, hit the scales at just 62kg and measured 1.74m tall compared to, say, Nairo Quintana, who weighs 58kg but is 7cm shorter. Where the general diets now vary is that riders will consume foods appropriate to the intensity of riding and time of year depending on the goals: that could be to lose weight, strengthen immunity (winter) or to pack glycogen levels ready for racing. In the past, as Hinault has commented, 'it was all about pasta and cereal'. Now, when it comes to general diets, fats are in. As for carbohydrates, they're still king in a race build-up and race situation. And you can find out more about that in Chapter 9.

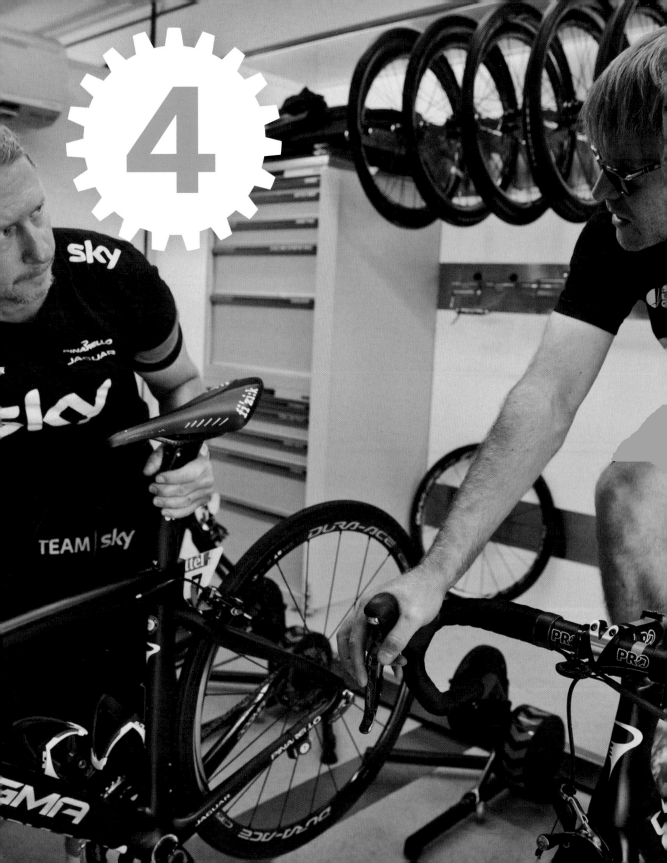

# TRAINING FOR THE TOUR

**The Tour de France features 22 teams** from across the globe with 17 of those coming from the WorldTour, which is the first division of cycling, the elite pinnacle of the sport. It guarantees you entrance to the world's most prestigious bike race. That leaves five spaces to fill, which comes down to the wildcard system – a discretionary selection from race organisers ASO. Teams are chosen from the 'second division' of professional cycling or the UCI Professional Continental level. It's the same template for the Giro d'Italia and La Vuelta, with the majority of wildcard spots filled by teams from the home nation. At the 2015 Tour, there were three French (Cofidis, Bretagne-Seche Environment and Thomas Voeckler's Europcar), one German (Bora-Argon 18) and one African (MTN-Qhubeka).

UCI rules state that each Tour team must comprise nine riders, who are supported by the manager, *directeurs sportifs*, trainers, doctors, therapists, soigneurs and mechanics. Added to that are the relatively new, but increasingly important, roles of head of sports science or simply sports scientist. And it's the interaction between sports scientist, trainer and rider that's vital because each rider will fulfil different roles, whether it's aiming for GC like Team Sky's Chris Froome, the sprint jersey in the style of André Greipel (Lotto-Soudal) or the king of the mountains like Rafał Majka (Tinkoff Sport).

## POSITION-SPECIFIC TRAINING

'We train for specific positions,' says Tinkoff Sport's former head of sports science Daniel Healey. 'But, though they're important, it's not just a case of telling the rider to look at the power meter and get on with it. Data is important but so is rider feedback. And that's where the coach comes in. They have to interpret both of those variables to prescribe the correct training. It's a neat cycling triangle.'

During periods of training, Healey and his team analyse the past week's sessions and then give the rider feedback every Monday morning. It's the summary

◁ Mechanics for Team Sky on a rest day at the 2014 Tour de France

of the week just gone and is the basis for what happens the following week. But, says David Martin of the Australian Institute of Sport, imparting this information and dictating what training a rider who might have 15 years of professional racing behind him will do next is more complex than you'd think.

'For years you've had a trainer and rider planning sessions,' says exercise physiologist Martin. 'Then a sports scientist comes up and says he can help you race faster. But how you communicate this message is important. I'll give you an analogy. Let's say you have a sophisticated software package to improve your chess. You're only used to moving pawns [for the first move] but, from reading the "help" scrolldown, you're told there's a strong move of the knight to the middle of the table. You've never done that before but you give it a go.

'I counter this with a move that puts pressure on your knight. You're not used to this because you've never opened with a knight before. I then take your knight and you're looking at this analytical package thinking, "Powerful? My ass. I've just lost my knight here". The problem is you don't know how to use it properly and that's because the expert who taught you how to use the software is a bit geeky, feels pressure from his job and says you're overcomplicating his instructions. This leaves you finding the whole experience ridiculously irritating.

'Or I could give you an attractive, calm woman who's easy to connect with and uses that voice in *Space Odyssey*. She doesn't give you more information than you need and also gives you a couple of options. You're in control but have guidance. Basically, how a sports scientist connects with coaches and riders is vital for performance.'

# COMPLEXITY OF THE LEAD-OUT

Ultimately cycling is a team sport, and how you communicate and react to others plays a huge part in whether you win or lose. That's not only between the support staff and riders, but also between the riders themselves. Clearly, those channels of communication and team spirit were at a peak when Mark Cavendish raced for the HTC-Highroad team. Before Cavendish moved to Team Sky at the end of 2011, leading to the HTC team's closure that same year, the men's and women's squads had accumulated a staggering 484 victories in four years, of which 30 were racked up by Cavendish at Grand Tours. HTC reset the sprinting benchmark of what was thought possible.

Time after time, his lead-out train delivered the Manx Missile to the front, at exactly the right time for Cavendish to do the rest. 'The stronger you are as a unit, the more you can control the race,' Cavendish told the BBC before the 2015 edition where he raced for Etixx–Quick-Step and won stage seven between Livarot and Fougères.

The lead-out is a complex organism and a previous good example was seen within Giant-Alpecin. Within the ranks of the German-licensed team were Marcel

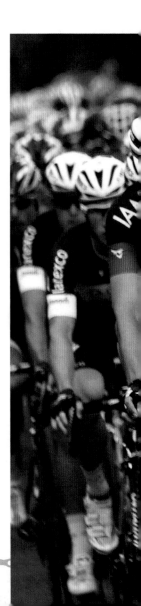

▽ Marcel Kittel used to be part of Giant-Alpecin's pure lead-out formation

Kittel and John Degenkolb – two of the strongest sprinters in the peloton but with markedly different characteristics.

'Marcel can generate incredibly high power output for a shorter period of time, while John, though a little less explosive, can still produce a strong sprint after 200km of hard racing,' says sports scientist at Giant-Alpecin Teun van Erp. 'If the race is 100–150km long and pretty flat, Marcel will always win but John has the ability to conserve power on the longest stages. I examined their power data when each of them hits top five, and if the race is longer and harder, John's performance goes up.'

Van Erp and his team took on-board the two markedly different characteristics and composed two different lead-out trains for the 2014 Tour de France, which they split into two categories: 'pure formation' for Marcel and his flat, all-out sprints, and 'power formation' for John, where the finish may be slightly uphill or feature a

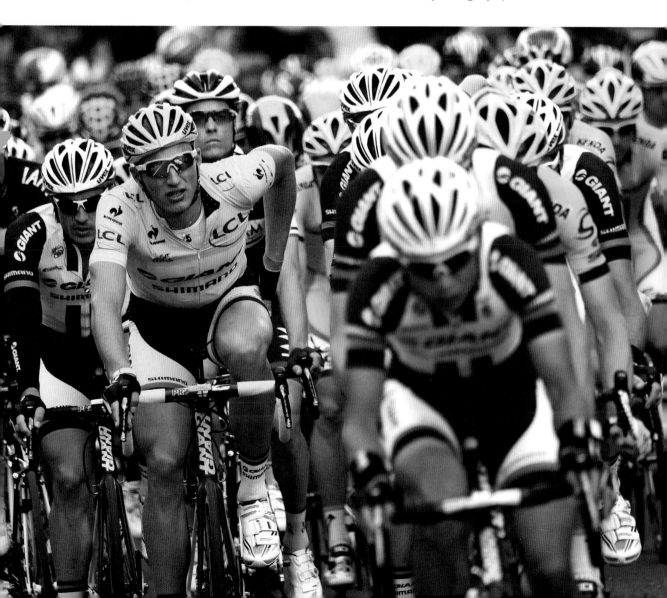

late climb. While the more controlled environment of the pure formation featured all nine riders, the more erratic nature of the power formation would theoretically comprise six riders.

Each of the riders was given a role with Giant's pure formation rolling out: Marcel Kittel, sprinter; Tom Veelers, lead-out; John Degenkolb, accelerator pilot; Koen de Kort, speed pilot; Roy Curvers, captain; Albert Timmer and Tom Dumoulin, positioners; Dries Devenyns and Cheng Ji, controllers.

It sounds like something out of a Thunderbirds film but each role is integral to, in the case of the pure formation, playing to Kittel's strengths. Let's begin with the controllers – their job starts early on. They try and take control of the stage, letting a breakaway go if there are no more than six or seven riders and they don't include riders from the other teams who are in sprint contention. Before the stage, the team would have calculated what would be a comfortable gap to let the break go, before slowly increasing the tempo to reel them in.

With the breakaway in their sights, the positioners will start to bring their team toward the front of the chasing pack. They'll crank up the pace and take 1km or 2km turns upfront. With around 1.5km before the finish line, it's time for the speed pilot to take charge. They'll put in an all-out 500m effort to either increase pace at the head of the pack or bring the team to the front. It's then up to the accelerator pilot to drive on again from 1km to 500m, ensuring pace is high enough to be in contention but ensuring the sprinter and lead-out don't lose his back wheel.

The lead-out sprints from around 600m to around 150m–250m depending on speed and wind direction. A headwind will see Kittel shelter behind Veelers that bit longer; a tailwind will see the big German open up earlier. Then it's showtime – over to the sprinter, who requires instinct and a cool demeanour to execute a winning finish. There's also the captain, who's like a composer, organising the team throughout the stage and being fully aware of what's going on. Experience is vital here.

It certainly worked for Giant-Alpecin, Kittel winning four times in 2014 to add to the quartet of stage wins the year before. 'We practise a lot in training,' says van Erp. 'There's a strong focus on maintaining high power outputs for many members of the team and particularly high wattage for the last two minutes of a stage. There's always a plan and every rider knows their responsibilities, though it's obviously such a frantic environment that you have to be flexible.'

Sprint training begins back in December where new sprint riders are introduced to the team with intensity of efforts picking up in January in time for the new season. Koen de Kort's been at the heart of the Giant lead-out train since 2009 and is finely tuned into the specificity and training of each role. 'I need high average power output for a decent amount of time – around 20–30 seconds – so that's what I train for,' he says. 'My training will differ to Marcel's because he needs maximum power for a very short period of time. I don't often train maximum power but a high

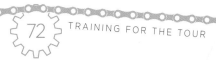

average power for a set period.

'For instance, during our training camp in Sierra Nevada before the 2015 Tour de France, Marcel [who didn't race in the end], John and I played a game where one would lead-out and the other two would sprint. Those two would beat me every time but when they stopped, I sprinted on for a longer period of time.'

Planning the lead-out train is a meticulous process. However, executing what you've practised in training within a race is far more unpredictable. The time trial is a solo challenge against the clock; hills leave the 198 riders spread out across slopes that can stretch for around 20km like the climbs of the Col d'Izoard and Ventoux; the sprint is different. Here, huge numbers of riders are penned in between temporary barriers and sponsors' billboards, reaching speeds of up to 50mph. It's no wonder crashes are a common occurrence and why the best place to train for the sprints is in the races.

'It's really hard to practise lead-outs in training because you can never replicate the stressful atmosphere of a race,' says Kittel. 'Teams are bumping into each other and fighting for space. That's why races leading into the Tour are so important.'

And why February races like the Tours of Qatar, Dubai and Oman are so important to teams aiming for sprint honours or the green jersey at the Tour. 'You learn a lot at those races,' says van Erp. 'At Dubai, for instance, we might not have got the results we were after but we learnt a lot about the dynamics of the lead-out.'

# PERIODISATION OF TRAINING

A team's build-up for the Tour de France usually begins in November the previous year. That's when the teams, who've often finished their season at October's Tour of Lombardy, regroup and set out plans for riders and the team, and subsequent training sessions.

'If you're a guy who's there for the sprints, we'll start them off with sprint work in December,' says Healey of Tinkoff Sport. 'But we do sprint work that doesn't compromise the aerobic work that we're doing. So as long as you keep the sprints short and do them from a rolling start, you can activate the neural system without producing too much lactate, so won't have detrimental effects on the other work you're doing at the time.'

Tradition says that you keep the intensity lower in the early winter months, before cranking things up in the New Year. But research suggests that's to neglect the importance of the nervous system on cycling performance, which is broken down into the central nervous system (brain and spinal cord) and peripheral nervous system, comprising cranial and spinal nerves. Every pedal stroke generated by Contador and Froome derives from the nervous system, and research indicates that prolonged and specific movement influences how the central nervous system controls muscle reactions.

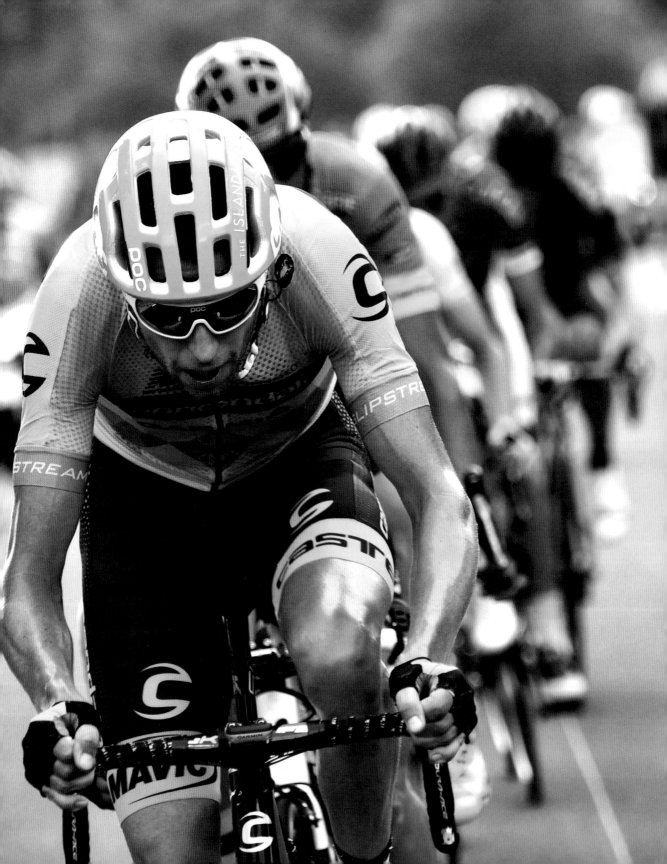

▽ Trek-Segafredo's Ryder Hesjedal (formerly Cannondale-Garmin) often builds his season around peaking at the Tour de France

Noted American coach Tudor Bompa examined the notion of 'receptors' and 'effectors' in weight training. Receptors are the stimuli and where you collect information, like the eyes and ears, while the effectors are the muscles that carry out the body's response to the stimuli. Bompa noted that to move the body as fast as possible when sprinting, the speed of signal transference in the central nervous system needed to be as rapid as possible, concluding that an athlete's receptors and effectors must be optimally excited and uninhibited for optimum recruitment of fast-twitch muscle fibres. In essence, by throwing in sprints on top of the aerobic week, Healey was reminding Sagan's central nervous system how to transfer a signal at fibre-optic speed. Leave out sprints from October to, say, February and your central nervous system could simply forget how to pedal fast!

'There's a very important cut-off point of no more than 10 seconds at that early part of the training year,' adds Healey. 'Up to that point you're producing energy from the ATP-PC system, which means you're not only engaging your brain with your short-term energy supply, but also not producing energy from carbohydrates, which would produce lactic acid and fatigue and that isn't what you want that early in the year. I'll tell them to go and have some fun, so do 5 seconds on, recover, 10 seconds on, and do that three or four times and vary the recovery time. Ultimately, sprinters want to sprint – it's what they do.'

Tinkoff Sport sprinters will also do these early off-season sprints from a rolling start – in other words, they'll build speed up gradually – so that they don't strain their muscles and potentially cause injury. They gradually increase the distances as the off-season progresses.

Compare this with Michael Rogers whose role is to protect and lead Alberto Contador at the major Tours. 'My role is quite different in the fact that when I'm working on a climb, it's up around threshold level (see Chapter 1), so below and above threshold and just holding that for a long time rather than all-out sprints. I also climb far more in training than someone like Sagan, who'd work on that top-end power for accelerations, and the more punchier riders.'

Healey's off-season sprint work with the likes of Sagan is an example of how training professional riders has evolved over the past few years. In the past, cyclists would spend the majority of the season racing, before having a brief holiday. On their return to training in November, they'd enter into what is now termed a 'traditional periodisation' model. Simplistically, this is where riders would build their stamina during the winter via long, mid-effort rides before upping the intensity as the race season approached. They'd hone speed at minor races, perhaps peaking for the cobbled or Ardennes classics in March and April before easing off slightly in preparation for the Tour so they'd hopefully peak come early July. In short, they'd build volume and then intensity.

Then along came Team Sky and Tim Kerrison who turned things on its head. Kerrison had arrived in Britain from Australian swimming where the concept of reverse periodisation was nothing new. So he started using that for cycling. Reverse periodisation is where instead of starting with volume in the winter, the rider focused on introducing power and speed from the start, before increasing the duration of the sessions as race season neared.

It's a periodisation model that requires a high aerobic base, which is something you see in elite cyclists. It also requires a stripped-down race schedule so that the rider can train themselves to peak rather than the old-school method of racing into fitness. And it's often attributed as one of the reasons why Team Sky can ride long periods at high tempo.

'Reverse periodisation is an interesting one,' says David Bailey, sports scientist at BMC Racing. 'All Tim did was say perhaps we don't need to do as much as we were doing. Tradition often drives things and that's especially true in cycling. That said, reverse by definition is probably wrong – you accumulate adaptations over years. From research and experience, if elites have a good, solid three or four years of training history, they don't need to build the same endurance base each winter. Your body becomes more efficient at responding to the training stimulus.'

Reverse periodisation demands more of the rider, though that extra intensity is offset with fewer races and a greater understanding of fatigue management (see Chapter 10 for more). As for Healey and his Tinkoff Sport team, 'I believe in the traditional model of periodised training with a few adjustments. I'm not going to tell you what these adjustments are, but they borrow from small pieces of the reverse periodisation model.'

Professional teams are notoriously guarded about their training cycles and composition, but an increasing body of evidence suggests that *block periodisation* could be the future (if not the present). 'A major limitation of the traditional periodisation model is its inability to produce multiple performance peaks over the season,' explains Iñigo Mujika, one of the world's leading sports scientists who formerly coached the now disbanded Euskaltel-Euskadi. 'When multiple races are closer together, riders need to extend their fitness peak, instead of trying to achieve a new peak for each race. That's where block periodisation comes in – it has the potential to extend your fitness peak.'

Block periodisation is a complex model, but essentially the rider works on specific fitness or technique goals in smaller chunks of time with occasional 'maintenance sessions' retaining the fitness gains from the previous block. As an example, the sports scientist who invented block periodisation, Vladimir Issurin, suggests the gains from aerobic endurance work, strength work and some form of technique – for example, refining pedal technique – might last between 25 and 35 days; anaerobic and muscular endurance work 15–23 days; and top-end gains, like maximum power output, five days.

With block training, the specific focus on, for example, speed will see the close proximity of speed sessions to the goal race elicit greater physical and biological changes than the traditional periodisation model, which will reward the high-end athlete with greater gains.

It's a complex model but one that was clarified by research from Bent Ronnestad of Lillehammer University in 2012. Ronnestad took two groups of highly trained cyclists and, over a four-week programme, made the riders perform eight high- and low-intensity training sessions. However, they spread these out differently – the block group undertook five high-intensity sessions in week one

## Periodisation of perfection

○ There are several different methods of determining a rider's training plan to reach peak performance. This is known as periodisation of training.

The top graph shows the traditional model of periodisation where the rider will work on general conditioning in the winter, move onto specific work (like speed) in the spring and then taper off to peak by the main races, like the Tour de France, before recovering.

The second graph is the block periodisation model, which features numerous smaller blocks of time, working on specific variables (like more power or speed), and is useful if you're looking to peak several times a season. This is becoming more common in the professional peloton.

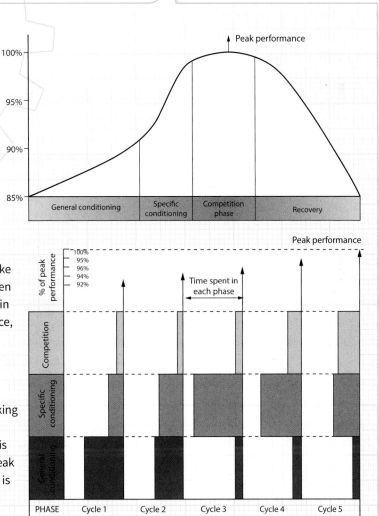

followed by three weeks of one high-intensity session compared to the traditional periodisation group's two high-intensity sessions per week. The study concluded that the block group exhibited a 4.6 per cent improvement in $VO_2$ max, a 2.1 per cent quicker time-trial effort and a 10 per cent increase in power output over the subjects following the traditional periodisation model. In short, the more intense blocks of high-intensity training led to fitness gains that eclipsed those of the traditional model.

Bailey uses block periodisation at BMC Racing but notes that its application varies rider by rider, trainer by trainer. As does Josu Larrazabal, trainer at Trek-Segafredo. 'It's not easy to speak in a few words about periodisation without being simplistic,' he says. 'We follow block periodisation but with interval training from the beginning. People who speak about "reverse" periodisation, they assume that's the only model where you have high-intensity training from the beginning, but we also apply intense sessions early in the training cycle but then increase their duration progressively like you would in the traditional model.'

'Ultimately, whatever model you choose, because of injury and illness it is the ability to remain flexible while compartmentalising training (thinking in terms of periodised blocks) that is key at this level,' says Healey. 'In my head I keep it really simple: you have to make the athlete fit, then strong, then powerful and then fast. That right there is a watered-down periodised model. The workouts you develop for each of these competencies is the real key and is very sensitive intellectual property.'

Despite the highly structured training plan, that doesn't mean each and every rider spends 364 days a year living within the confines of the team. Most teams run three to five training camps a year, varying from one to two weeks. The riders then spend race time with the team, meaning they're away from home for around 150 days each year. They're expected to follow the training protocol when at home, and as their livelihood and stardom depends on it, it's rare you'll find a cyclist turn up to training camp and receiving a rollicking for piling on the pounds.

# SQUATTING POWER

It's not just on-the-bike training that's undergone a makeover – what cyclists do off the bike is changing, too. 'In the winter I spend a lot of time in the gym,' says multiple green-jersey winner Peter Sagan. 'I'm mainly working on my legs. The squat is very important.' Kittel mirrors Sagan's gym training. 'In the winter I'm really busy in the gym, doing a lot of squats – around 120kg – and core workouts,' he says. 'The focus then is on high weights and low repetitions to build power output. In the summer, weight sessions are less frequent and the workouts comprise lower weights and more repetitions. This adds sustainability to your sprints.'

'The other aspect of training we're looking at is tailor-made weight-training programmes to satisfy the needs of the individual rider,' says Etixx–Quick-Step coach Peter Hespel. 'The types of weight training you need for a hill climber, or a Cavendish, or Tom Boonen is different. You have to do different types of resistance training because nobody has ever won the Tour based on explosive strength – you win it on the time trials and the mountain stages.'

Much of this focus on the gym by WorldTour teams is down to a 2010 journal article by Per Aagaard and Jesper Andersen who examined the effect of strength training on endurance capacity in top-level endurance athletes. After poring over years' worth of studies, the researchers concluded that strength training can lead to endurance, power and strength benefits for highly trained cyclists, especially, though not exclusively, by employing a high-volume, high-resistance weight protocol.

> You have to make the athlete fit, then strong, then powerful and then fast.
>
> **Daniel HEALEY,** *Tinkoff Sport*

'Everyone in this team does off-season weight training – the sprinter, climber, rouleur,' says Healey. 'When you weight train, you lay a big bed of muscle fibres that helps to soak up lactic acid as the intensity of riding rises. That can give you up to a 6 per cent increase in threshold for free as opposed to simply riding. There's irrefutable evidence that it works all-year round but sadly it's impractical – we'd need an extra bus decked out with the gym equipment we'd need for the guys to strength train.'

It's interesting to note that Healey cites facilities rather than time of year as the reason weight training ends as tradition suggests it's weight-derived muscle damage – and how that would reduce the effectiveness of the next session – that stops riders from hitting the gym in race season. It's also interesting to note how Kittel and Sagan both highlighted the importance of squats.

'Your quadriceps are integral to a powerful pedal stroke,' says Larrazabal. 'But other supporting muscles are, too. That's why squats are so useful. When you're standing with the bar on your shoulders, first you need to fix the position to give balance to your body or you can't do the movement. So you activate other muscles simply to keep you standing. That realistically simulates cycling where every movement requires muscles to fix the position, while others focus on generating power.'

But the sight of Cancellara and co. straining under 200kg with veins bursting out of their respective foreheads couldn't be further from the truth. While track riders will often be working to exhaustion using weights that could forge craters, the needs of Tour riders are very different. They're still looking for maximum strength, whether it's for an all-out sprint, fighting a headwind or ascending Alpe d'Huez, but that intense burst of effort will feature in an endurance-based ride of up to six hours.

'That's why it's all about the speed of the squat that's important, not necessarily the weight,' says Larrazabel. 'We use a device similar to a power meter on a bike that measures the speed of your squat called T-Force. With that knowledge, the number of reps almost becomes irrelevant – it's about holding the pace of the squat.'

'For the loads we're looking to use, ideally the riders are performing a full squat in 0.9m to 1.2m per second,' adds Larrazabel. 'If they do it faster than that, we increase the weight but it's never usually beyond 40 or 50kg. Key, though, is that we'll never take them past five or six repetitions as we're looking to "strengthen" the neuromuscular system rather than bulk up their muscles. It's taken the riders a while to adjust because they're a species that's used to suffering.'

Riccardo Colucci is a man mountain with biceps that resemble the Galibier. He's a former international swimmer, artistic gymnast, martial artist and now personal trainer. Tinkoff Sport hired the Italian to 'create riders that are more efficient and waste less energy'. Colucci achieves this lofty aim through core training – something that, unlike weights, WorldTour riders perform all-year round.

'I use very simple tools: sticks, resistance bands and the floor,' adds Colucci. 'The more simple, the more refined the intervention. The more complex the tool, the less the human body has to do. Plus it means they can do the exercises when they're staying in something like an Ibis at the Tour.'

At training camp, Tinkoff Sport riders undertake core training twice a day. Exercises like the plank are designed to strengthen your abdominal area and lower back, which are key muscle groups for a cyclist who'll be racing over 2,000 miles crouched over a carbon bike. The rest of the year, out of the gaze of the support staff, riders ideally do core work every day, though realism often kicks in. 'The past few years I've done the bare minimum,' says Michael Rogers of Tinkoff Sport. 'There's only 24 hours in the day. Between training and family, I find it hard to dedicate time to core, though I do a 15 min core session three to four times a week.'

Rogers is one of the few riders who doesn't do weights, either, 'not for the past 10 years anyway'. And when the season's over, he leaves the bike in the shed and begins … running. 'I run for up to an hour every third day and I love it,' he says. 'I've been doing it for years and I've discovered it's improved my peak power by 2 to 3 per cent. When you're cycling, your muscles are contracting and become scrunched up. Running lengthens them and gives them back their elasticity.'

Rogers notes that many of the riders in the peloton slip into running shoes before the bike training really picks up, though wisely off-road rather than joint-stressing tarmac. 'I've found that runners with skinny legs like me enjoy it. The muscular ones seem to struggle.'

As well as stretching their legs, it could also benefit power output, as Rogers described. The weight-bearing nature of running stimulates a greater testosterone release than cycling. This is down to micro-tears caused by the high impact of running, which stimulates a muscle-repairing process that requires testosterone. This is key to building strength and power. On the flipside, the higher impact means injury risk is higher so coaches advise cyclists to keep running to a minimum.

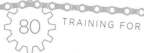

# Training plan

○ David Bailey is a sports scientist and performance coach at BMC Racing, whose roster includes Tejay van Garderen and Richie Porte. Here he reveals how a GC rider's weekly training plan varies depending on the season.

'This is a bit of a mix to give an insight into the different training sessions that might be included during these periods,' explains Bailey. 'Normally a GC rider focuses on one of those – for instance, time-trial work or aerobic capacity – for a given block of around three to four weeks in order to maximise the training effect. A week is normally a little long for a microcycle (small chunk of training plan with specific physiological aims) of this nature. Hence, you might find GC riders work on three- to four-day blocks.

'Finally, the "in-season" training week is literally in between races – Monday to Sunday. An "in season" training block in the build-up to races would look a little different with some race-specific work depending on the performance goal.'

| DAY | OFF-SEASON (WINTER) TRAINING | IN-SEASON TRAINING |
|---|---|---|
| **Monday** | 4-hour ride inc. low-cadence intervals: 2 × 4–6 × 4–8 minutes seated climbing <60rpm @ 50–60% functional threshold (FTP) | 2-hour easy post-race ride |
| **Tuesday** | 4-hour ride inc. time-trial intervals, intensity reaching FTP over 45–60 minutes with short and long efforts | 1-hour strength and conditioning gym session; day off bike |
| **Wednesday** | 5-hour ride inc. aerobic capacity effort intervals: 2 × 4–6 × 4–6 minutes @ 110–125% FTP, plus 20–30 variable-intensity climbing efforts | 3-hour time-trial intervals, intensity reaching FTP over 30–45 minutes with short and long efforts |
| **Thursday** | 3-hour easy ride plus strength and conditioning gym session | 5-hour endurance ride inc. 1–1.5 hours medium-intensity climbing |
| **Friday** | 6-hour endurance ride inc. 3–4 × 30–40 minutes of variable-intensity climbs | 3-hour easy ride but with 30–60 minutes motor pacing in the last hour |
| **Saturday** | 7-hour endurance ride inc. 1–1.5 hours of medium-intensity climbing plus 1 × 20–30 minutes variable-intensity climb in the last hour | 2-hour pre-race ride inc. 3 × 10 minutes medium-intensity efforts |
| **Sunday** | 1-hour strength and conditioning gym session; day off bike | 6-hour race day |

# TAPERING TO PEAK

Once the riders have racked up thousands of miles at different intensities, lifted weights, stretched out their lower back and even gone for a run, all that's left is for them is to peak for the Tour de France. Well, no. Clearly the world's greatest race is part of a schedule that might require peaking at the Classics and then the Tour or, in the case of Contador in 2015, the Giro and then the Tour. Ensuring you're at your best for your goal races, when you're competing for around 80–100 days each year, is a difficult proposition, but one attempted by coaches and riders through 'tapering', that is, tapering off amount or intensity of training.

When the riders are training, they're trading the fatigue of the session with the potential benefits of improving fitness. When it comes to peaking for the Tour, they want to clear out fatigue, leaving them fresher and, ideally, at peak fitness. Get the tapering process right and they could enjoy performance improvements over the pre-taper of 2–3 per cent – and that's down to a myriad of physiological changes. Studies have looked at the effects of tapering on blood parameters such as haemoglobin (oxygen-carrying capacity of red blood cells), haematocrit (percentage of red blood cells in the blood) and red blood cell volume (size of red blood cells). Mujika discovered all three rose in a taper.

Further research suggests tapering strengthens the contractile properties of muscle fibres, while white-blood cell count – and therefore immunity – rises. The aim of the taper is also to increase testosterone and reduce cortisol levels.

Studies have shown that optimal tapering duration for cycle racing ranges from between eight and 14 days, with training volume dropping by around 41–60 per cent by reducing either the duration or frequency of the sessions. However, maintaining intensity is a key factor in retaining or further increasing fitness adaptations during the taper. This is proven – but for one-day events only.

'How you freshen up for a three-week event is very different to a one-day event and is also different for nearly every team,' says David Martin. 'Firstly there's the altitude aspect, when they timed their pre-Tour camp and whether they might have raced at something like the Dauphiné or Tour of Switzerland.

'One example might be that the rider will have a really light week two weeks before a big race or Tour, throwing in the occasional quality session. But they'll focus on sleeping well and not travelling. Then a week out they'll throw in a couple of really big climbs so that they might not feel as fit as they can be for the start of the Tour but they feel ready. Come week two, they'll be growing stronger and then peaking for the final week.'

Michael Rogers again highlights the importance of TrainingPeaks as a tool

> If I start too fresh, my heart rate goes so high that my energy levels are depleted straight away.
>
> **Michael ROGERS,** *Tinkoff Sport*

that's taken the guesswork out of peaking. 'It's had a huge impact, especially if you have a lot of data,' he says, before revealing that feeling fresh for a three-week race isn't necessarily the aim for stage one. 'It's a good idea for me to start a race underdone rather than overdone. If I start too fresh, my heart rate goes so high that in those first few days, it's almost a double-edge sword and my energy levels are depleted straight away.'

Rogers highlights the difficulty of peaking for a 21-stage race – which is compounded by your race goal. A rider like Fabian Cancellara, for instance, would have been looking to peak for the opening prologue at the 2015 Tour de France whereas someone like Contador or Froome look to crank it up after nine or ten stages when the mountains come into view.

'Interestingly these guys train pretty hard up to the event,' says Cannondale-Garmin manager Jonathan Vaughters. 'With professional cyclists, the more they train, the more they have to train to retain homeostasis [i.e. their body in balance], so tapering isn't as important as it is at lower levels.'

There's a huge amount of theorising in search of standardising tapering and periodised models. Intervals will be shortened and recovery lengthened, and vice versa, in the search to unravel the complexity of making the human body higher, faster and stronger. Over to Vaughters. 'I've seen over and over again that guys who are good at three-week Tours, although their heart rate will be suppressed and they'll be showing other signs of fatigue from a haematological standpoint, their power output really doesn't drop at all.

'Yes, maybe for the occasional short effort but, for the real GC contender, holding power for longer can actually go up,' he continues. 'It's what happened to Ryder [Hesjedal] at the 2015 Giro when he finished fifth. His power was notice-ably higher in the final week. That's why we raced him more before heading to Italy because he's done it before where he comes into his own as the race continues. It worked – a bit.'

'There are many different types of talent in cycling,' adds Vaughters. 'Many focus on $VO_2$ but a better marker is how a rider adapts to high training load. That is a talent and some guys who might have much lower $VO_2$s might have a much higher capacity to adapt. Ryder has mediocre $VO_2$ but incredible ability to adapt to high workload. It's like Darwinism. If the rider can adapt, they'll go further.' Of course, that's not simply down to the human – increasingly, the machine is playing a significant role in how fast a rider can reach the finish line.

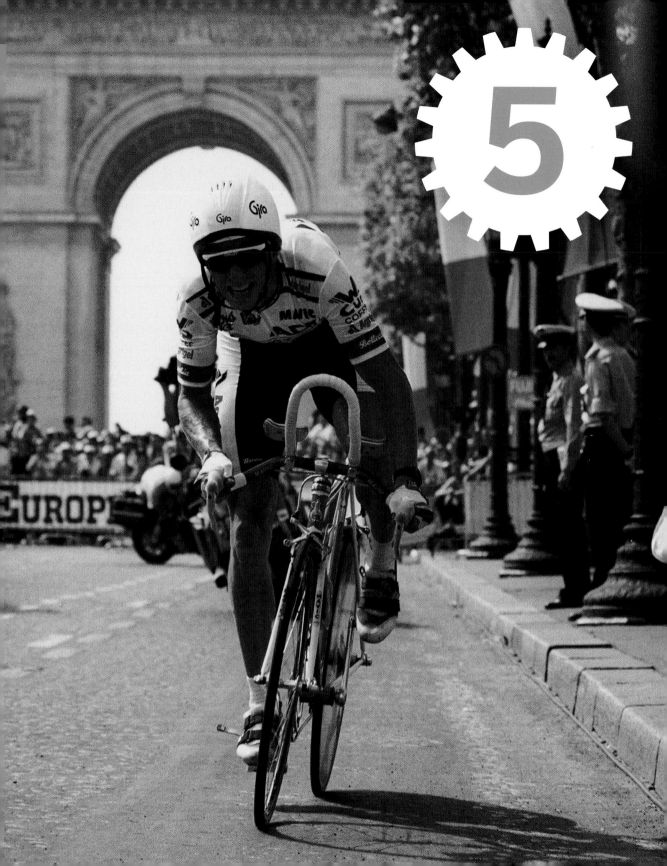

# BIKE & WHEEL INNOVATION

Over time, stage 21 of the 1989 Tour de France has cultivated mythical status, such is its Hollywood ending. At the start of the final stage and after 3,260km of racing, America's Greg LeMond trailed Laurent Fignon by 50 seconds. All that stood between home favourite Fignon and his third title was a short 24.5km time trial from Versailles to Paris. Such was the partisan confidence that French newspapers had prepared special editions with Fignon on the front page.

LeMond stepped out of the team bus and onto his bike, and looked like he'd landed from outer space. His head was covered with a sleek-looking helmet, while a pair of bar extensions borrowed from triathlon protruded from his cockpit. Fignon, on the other hand, followed tradition, racing without a helmet, leaving his long blonde ponytail flowing in the Parisian air. He also eased himself down onto traditional dropped handlebars rather than LeMond's futuristic platform.

LeMond rode at an average speed of 54.55km/h, at the time the fastest time trial ever ridden at the Tour. Fignon, his face tightening with every pedal stroke, gave his all down the Champs Élysées but it wasn't enough. He was 58 seconds slower than the American, giving LeMond victory by just 8 seconds – the smallest winning margin in the race's history. For many, that was the day the sport realised the impact that aerodynamics has on performance. (In fact, many speculated at the time that had Fignon chopped off his locks, he'd have won.)

Bikes have come a long way and the ones ridden by Fignon and LeMond were a far cry from the first Tour bikes that were constructed from heavy steel frames, wooden wheels and had only two gears, the rider having to flip the back wheel to shift up or down. These bikes could weigh up to 16kg and featured traditional round tubing.

Fast-forward to today's Tour de France and the bikes tip the scales at the 6.8kg mark, which is comparable with the carry-on weight limit of many airlines. They're also incredibly aerodynamic. A few weeks ahead of the 2015 Tour, Specialized whetted technophiles' appetites by unveiling Mark Cavendish's new S-Works Venge ViAS aero-dynamic road bike. Noises coming out of Specialized HQ in California suggested it was

◁ Greg LeMond famously employed cutting-edge aerodynamics to win the 1989 Tour de France two minutes faster than a standard road bike over a 40km time trial and one minute faster than the previous incarnation of the Venge. It certainly looked slick, with an aerodynamic stem housing the cabling, a rear brake built into the seat tube for aero-dynamic savings and mightily slender headtube giving it a minuscule frontal profile.

Then there's the 795 from French manufacturers Look, used by French team Bretagne-Séché Environnement at the 2015 Tour. The gently ascending top tube flows into the stem with the ease of Quintana ascending Alpe d'Huez; you can adjust the stem from 17° to −13° depending on your aero-dynamic bent.

'It also comes with or without integrated brakes, integrated routings and inte-grated seatpost,' says Look general manager Jean-Claude Chrétien. 'We're big on integration.' Hiding components behind frame and fork tubing is something manu-facturers are spending more time on with the goal of reducing drag and increasing free speed.

'They're starting to look like track bikes,' says Lotto-Soudal's Greg Henderson, who began his career on the track before moving to the road and now rides on Ridley bikes. 'And they're similarly fast.'

# TUBING REVOLUTION

Aerodynamic road bikes are all curves and concealment in search of more stream-lined speed. And you can see why when you understand the physics. 'As a cyclist you're faced with a number of resistive forces,' says Bert Blocken, professor of physics at Eindhoven University of Technology in the Netherlands. 'These are the rolling resis-tance of the tyres, friction in the chain and bearings, and the aerodynamic resistance to motion.' We give a further overview of how each of these forces affects the rider in Chapter 2 on bike fit. Here, we're looking at the aero-dynamic resistance because this provides the greatest barrier to Tour riders, the only exception potentially being at very slow speeds on very steep hills. In fact, at race speeds, aerodynamic drag of the bike and rider has been measured at 96 per cent of total resistance. So, anything the sports scientists can do to reduce the drag, the better.

Adorning our boffin's hat for just one moment, air resistance = 0.5 × air density × cycling speed (in still air) squared × the drag coefficient of the rider and bike × the frontal area of the rider and bike. (Again, you can find out more about the inter-action of these forces in Chapter 2.)

Professional teams can't do too much about air density when it comes to racing, though they maximise it when it comes to altitude training (see Chapter 7). It does highlight, however, why air temperature's so important when it comes to an event like the hour record. In the build-up to Bradley Wiggins' record-breaking attempt in June 2015, the 2012 Tour de France winner told reporters, 'Much of the hour record is dictated by temperature and air pressure. I'm not a weather man but if you have really low pressure – under 1,000 [grams per cubic metre] – you'll travel

## Weight watchers

○ **The following timeline** shows how advancements in material technology has seen bike weights drop over the past 50 years. Each entry shows the winner for that year, the bike manufacturer and the weight (lbs and kgs).

| | | |
|---|---|---|
| **1962** | Jacques **ANQUETIL**, *Helyett* | 22.4 (10.4) |
| **1965** | Felice **GIMONDI**, *Magni* | 24.2 (11) |
| **1972** | Eddy **MERCKX**, *Colnago* | 21.1 (9.6) |
| **1987** | Stephen **ROCHE**, *Battaglin* | 21.1 (9.6) |
| **1994** | Miguel **INDURAIN**, *Pinarello-badged (Dario Pegoretti)* | 19.8 (9.0) |
| **1998** | Marco **PANTANI**, *Bianchi* | 17.8 (8.1) |
| **2003** | Lance **ARMSTRONG**, *Trek 5900 SL* | 15.9 (7.2)* |
| **2006** | Oscar **PEREIRO**, *Pinarello Dogma-FPX* | 15.0 (6.8) |
| **2009** | Alberto **CONTADOR**, *Trek Madone 6-series* | 15.0 (6.8) |
| **2015** | Chris **FROOME**, *Pinarello Dogma F8* | 15.0 (6.8) |

\* Disqualified for doping, though the year before UCI brought in minimum weight regulations.

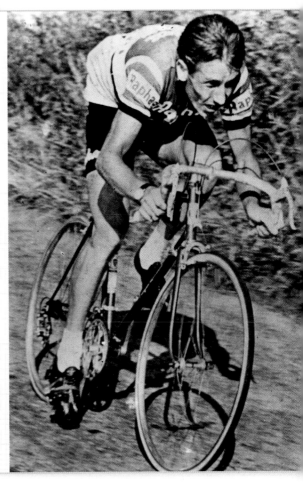

▷ Jacques Anquetil won five Tour titles on steel bikes

a lot further on the day; anything up to an extra 1km for the same power.' Warm air is also less dense than cold air. As it transpired, the barometric Gods were with Wiggins who rode 54.526km, surpassing Alex Dowsett's mark of 52.937km.

While the team at Lee Valley velodrome, home to the record attempt, controlled temperature at a constant 28°C inside the velodrome, out on the roads of France riders can't influence the weather conditions. However, the bike manufacturers and rider can influence the drag coefficient and frontal area parts of that aerodynamic equation.

'Drag is primarily down to two aspects for the cyclist,' explains Rob Lewis of CFD (computational fluid dynamics) specialists TotalSim, who've regularly worked with British Cycling. 'One is skin drag, which is the friction of the air rubbing over the surface. The other is pressure drag. That's harder to explain but, essentially, is why a brick has more drag than the same-sized object but in a more streamlined shape.'

A blunt, irregular object disturbs the air flowing around it, forcing the air to separate from the object's surface. Low-pressure regions from behind the object result in a pressure drag against the object. With high pressure in the front and low pressure behind, the cyclist is literally being pulled backwards.

It's why tubing is at the forefront of this frame revolution with teardrop shaping, or variant of, a popular choice. 'The difference between round tubing and streamlined tubing goes back to the 1950s,' says Lewis. 'Professor Ascher Shapiro [one-time professor of mechanical engineering at MIT] showed that airflow is far more turbulent passing over round objects compared to a smooth airfoil, which is essentially a tapered tube.'

Teardrop-shaping formed the basis of nearly every bike at the 2015 Tour. You can see it on the Cervélo S5 that sat beneath the chamois pads of MTN-Qhubeka riders like Steve Cummings, who won stage 14, and Edvald Boasson Hagen; Andre Greipel rode the teardrop-shaped Ridley Noah SL to four victories; and the 'flattened' teardrop tubing can be seen on Chris Froome's Pinarello Dogma F8. So what exactly is it about this teardrop tubing that slips through the air like Kittel through the peloton?

'It's down to the coefficient of drag,' explains Simon Smart, who helped design the original Giant Trinity and Scott's Plasma and Foil bikes. The coefficient of drag is a dimensionless quantity that is used to measure the drag or resistance of an object in a fluid environment such as air or water. 'For a cylinder, coefficient of drag measures one,' Smart continues. 'But a teardrop wing section of the same diameter can have a value of 0.05, which is a 20th of the drag of a cylinder.'

'You have what's called a bluff body where the flow can't stay streamlined and attached, particularly on a cylinder or a wire,' Smart continues. 'The flow just goes around the front to the maximum width, before separating and creating a lot of pressure behind the rider. That's bluff body aerodynamics.' For an illustrative example of Smart's words, see the 'Teardrop tubing' box, on page 90.

With the drag of a cylinder 20 times more than a teardrop shape, you could have a cylinder that's 10mm wide and it'll create the same drag as an airfoil shape that's 200mm wide. 'There's a huge advantage of tapering a shape so the air can flow around it and then recover,' adds Smart. 'That's what our aerodynamics is about.'

A teardrop shape keeps what's termed a laminar boundary attached to its surface longer than a cylindrical tube, whose round shape creates mini vortices because of the pressure differential, which increases drag. It begs the question: if this airfoil shape becomes more aerodynamic the greater the ratio between its width and depth, why don't bike manufacturers create efforts like the Lotus superbike, which featured such large fairings that it resembled a sail and propelled Chris Boardman to Olympic gold in 1992?

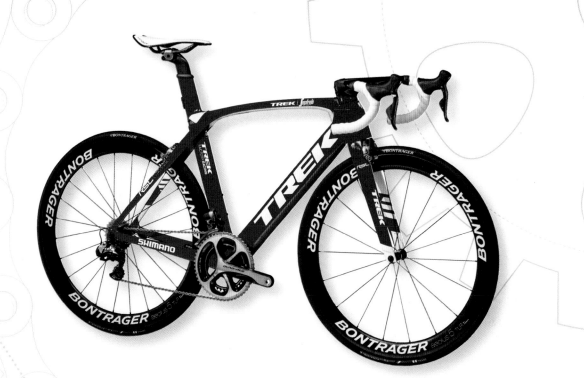

# RESTRAINED BY THE UCI

△ Trek's Madone 9 utilises Kammtail Virtual Foil tubing for increased aerodynamics

'For a start, there's a tipping point where a higher-aspect ratio becomes less efficient,' says Smart. 'Reach something like 7:1 (where the depth of the frame tubing is seven times greater than the width) and it starts to lose momentum because of how the air flows at low speed.'

But the primary reason is because of the UCI (cycling's international governing body) and their lengthy regulations. Regarding equipment, the UCI rules state: 'The enforcement of the rules improves fairness and safety during the races: limit the impact of the equipment on the performance; the race victory to the best rider, not the best machine; the preservation of the culture and image of the bicycle …'

The aim is to prevent cycling morphing into Formula One, which in popular opinion has shifted to more about the car's ability than the driver's. When it comes to airfoil shape, the UCI states that the ratio must not exceed 3:1 'for the frame, fork, handlebars, extensions, stem and seatpost'.

It's a bone of contention amongst many bike manufacturers who feel the 3:1 regulation restricts innovation. Bike designers are an innovative lot, mind you, and have come up with a multitude of ways to try and enjoy greater aerodynamic effects without upsetting the UCI.

'As part of our ongoing development of aerodynamic bikes, we utilised the Kammtail technology that was originally developed for automotive use,' says Trek engineer Doug Cusack, whose 2015 Madone 9 employs this shaping for their tubing.

Trek first introduced this aerodynamic phenomenon to their Speed Concept range in 2010. The American giants used 5:1 airfoil tubing, before slicing off the end to create an actual 3:1 shape but the airflow purportedly still reacting as it would with the 5:1 tubing.

'When air flows over a truncated aerodynamic shape, it fills in the missing tail with a recurring vortex of air that takes the shape of a virtual tail,' continues Cusack. 'It gives the truncated shape with drag almost as low as a full deep-section airfoil. An interesting side benefit is that at the speeds that a bicycle travels, the virtual tail changes shape to allow for even more efficient airflow by allowing the tail to bend to the most efficient shape as the angle of the wind flow changes.'

How much further bike manufacturers can play around with that teardrop shaping remains to be seen but things could be set to change. In September 2015,

## Teardrop tubing

The diagram below shows how Trek's Kammtail technology, as seen on their bikes like the Madone 9, purports to reduce the separation of air from the tubing and create less of a turbulent wake. UCI regulations stipulate that tubing can't be greater than a 3:1 ratio; in other words, the tubing can't be three times longer than it is wide. Around 6–7:1 ratio is the optimum streamlined shape without too great a weight penalty. Trek overcame this 3:1 limitation by designing a tube that's 5:1 in proportion and then carving the end off to keep within the 3:1 parameters. The illustration shows how this improves aerodynamics when the wind is coming at the rider from 10°. Trek say this blunting of the tubes amounts to a 25-watt saving.

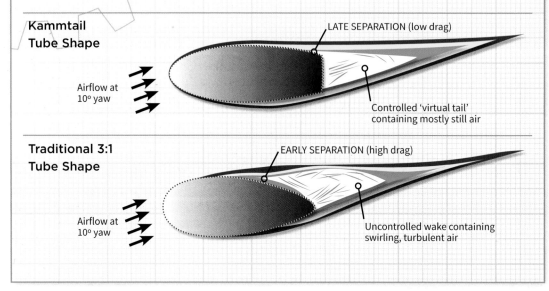

**Kammtail Tube Shape**

Airflow at 10° yaw

LATE SEPARATION (low drag)

Controlled 'virtual tail' containing mostly still air

**Traditional 3:1 Tube Shape**

Airflow at 10° yaw

EARLY SEPARATION (high drag)

Uncontrolled wake containing swirling, turbulent air

## The 6.8kg rule

○ Every sport has a numerical figure (or figures) that resonates for many. In English football it's 1966, in American football it's 49 (San Francisco) and in golf it's 1 (the number of shots all golfers dream of ticking off a par three). In cycling it's 6.8 – or it has been since 2000.

That's when the Lugano Charter was officially sanctioned by the UCI (cycling's governing body), bringing in a host of regulations designed to uphold a rather noble ideal: that cycling should be a sport of athletes, not machine. The 3:1 rule (see the 'Teardrop tubing' box on page 90) was brought in to limit the impact of aerodynamics, efforts by Chris Boardman and Graeme Obree cited as steeds that were simply too shapely, too fast and focused more on machine than man.

The UCI also brought in a rule stating that bikes should weigh more than the rather arbitrary figure of 6.8kg. The reasoning was sound with the UCI stating that any less than this could threaten the structure of the bike and make it unsafe. But times and materials move on and, as UCI president Brian Cookson recently admitted, 'I understand why the rule was brought in, though I think the technology has moved on.' The industry is keen to lower the limit – lighter is always a good selling point to the masses – and though a limit is necessary to maintain safety standards, it seems inevitable that the UCI will lower the limit in the future. The UCI aren't ones for succumbing to pressure, though, so whether that'll be in 2017 or 2027 remains to be seen.

the bicycle committee of the World Federation Sporting Goods Industry (WFSGI) was charged with working with the UCI to change the rules on that 3:1 tube limitation as well as the 6.8kg minimum weight (see above). It's a far cry from the 1990s when two engineers were free to transform the world of bike aerodynamics.

# CERVÉLO – AERODYNAMIC INNOVATORS

Over 20 years ago, professor Ascher Shapiro's airflow observations filtered through to Eindhoven where engineering student Gerard Vroomen began researching bike dynamics. He continued his research at McGill University, Canada, before meeting fellow engineer and cycle nut Phil White. In 1995, the two of them founded Cervélo Cycles and set to work on creating some of the most groundbreaking – but, more importantly, aerodynamic – bikes the world had seen.

One of the first bikes to come out of Cervélo was in 1995 when White and Vroomen designed and built a time-trial bike for double world champion Gianni Bugno. The famous green steed featured no discernible seat stay or downtube; instead, the curvaceous number consisted primarily of an extra-long and deep seat tube that flowed into a top tube that hugged the front wheel. Its cutting-edge design reportedly delighted Bugno. His sponsors didn't receive the bike with equally open arms, thinking its design was too extreme to appeal to the conservative consumer, and he never rode it in competition. While Bugno's Cervélo never went to market, White and Vroomen learnt a huge amount about aerodynamics.

'The very first Cervélo we designed, the airfoil shapes came from NACA, which was predecessor of NASA,' says Vroomen, who sold his stake in Cervélo in 2011 to pursue new ventures in mountain biking. 'We undertook a helluva lot of research on patterns of airflow at different speeds and their characteristics. We looked at the NACA book, slapped them onto the frames and tested them against the competition of the time. All of them were faster, which isn't surprising as we were competing against round tubes. We were miles ahead.'

Cervélo also became one of the first bike manufacturers to regularly use the wind tunnel. 'When we started out, we used a thin steel frame that we could clad with plastic covers (aero shapes). By having a very thin steel frame, we had the structural integrity to add the shapes, which we could move around depending on what data was coming back. We could put a mannequin on; in fact, we could even put a person on it.'

Wind tunnels used to be the preserve of the aviation and motor industry with the poorer siblings from the bike industry relying on hire time. Though hire time is still the norm, Specialized became the first manufacturer to build an in-house tunnel in 2013, and the Flanders government has also invested €500,000 in a facility that will be used by several companies including Ridley and Lazer.

'Wind tunnels are an invaluable tool,' says Damon Rinard, engineer at Cannondale who used to work with Cervélo. 'You can use the same mannequin on each bike; the same fit coordinates for each bike; isolate the variable in question – frame, forks, wheels.'

In short, they give data and that's what engineers thrive on to progress. Mark Spore is an engineer for BAE Systems and has worked in wind tunnels for years in Preston, England, predominantly testing aircraft and missiles. In 2010 he partnered with UK Sport, testing a number of different GB track cycling athletes in the build-up to the London Games. 'They came along with their own equipment and we projected drag information onto the floor in front of them,' says Spore. 'They then changed their position to see the drag effect. Athlete positioning, gear and clothing all had an impact … but the results are sensitive so I can't say more than that.'

The next evolutionary leap revolved around the use of computational fluid dynamics (CFD). It's a computer-based tool that studies fluids, including gases, and the forces on them. Through numerical methods and algorithms, computers can accurately determine the airflow on and around an object. So if you want to find out the drag on a specific shape of tubing and how it interacts with the rider and wheels, you simply program the details into CFD and await the results. Not only is this method cheaper than wind-tunnel use, it's also highly accurate, results coming in within 1.5 per cent of real-world performance.

'It was great to use the tunnel but damn expensive,' says Vroomen. 'It used to come in at around $1,000 an hour. Thankfully CFD came along and made things a lot cheaper. Mind you, it was a lot harder to master CFD for cycling than for aerospace and automotive. Think of a car. It's a body with four small wheels. On a bike, nearly everything is moving. A car is child's play. Grown-ups work on bikes.'

So while manufacturers continue to hire and use wind tunnels, unless you're Specialized who has their own, they're increasingly used as a validation tool rather than a design one. And that's part of the reason why aerodynamics is spreading to other parts of the riding package – with R&D costs reduced, you can apply aero research into, say, overshoes that wouldn't have been financially viable in a tunnel. (For more information, see the next chapter, which focuses on components and apparel.)

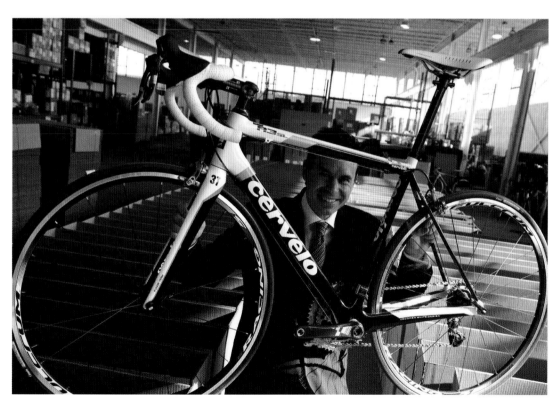

# How aero at the Tour?

○ German bike magazine *Tour* is acclaimed as providing the most thorough bike tests of any magazine on the market. That's because they take each bike into the wind tunnel, testing the frame with its own wheelset and, for comparative purposes, with Zipp's 404 Firecrest.

The graph shows the measured watt values of five aerodynamic road bikes that featured at the 2015 Tour de France and the absolute ride times they result in – both with original wheels and mounted with Zipp 404s – over a 62-mile route that comprised 2,000m of climbing. The simulation takes into account aerodynamics and weight, assuming a constant pedalling of 200 watts with the rider in a static, brake-grip holding position, a rider weight of 75kg, original weights for the bike and wheels, and assumes no slipstreaming.

The fastest bikes are the Cervélo S5 and Canyon Aeroroad CF SLX 9.0 LTD, which both achieve a riding time of 4 hours, 15 minutes and 29 seconds.

**Aerodynamic advantages expressed in absolute times**

| Model | Ride time in hours and minutes |
|---|---|
| CERVÉLO S5 Dura-Ace | 4:15:28 (205W) |
| | 4:15:35 (210W) |
| CANYON Aeroad CF SLX 9.0 LTD | 4:15:29 (210W) |
| | 4:15:29 (230W) |
| GIANT Propel Advanced SL | 4:15:51 (212W) |
| | 4:15:51 (212W) |
| SPECIALIZED S-Works Venge Dura-Ace | 4:16:03 (216W) |
| | 4:15:49 (213W) |
| MERIDA Reacto Team-E | 4:16:52 (206W) |
| | 4:16:11 (212W) |

Original wheelset

Zipp 404 Firecast wheels

# CARBON REFINEMENT

Manufacturers continue to innovate. Tubes are being made more slippery and anything that used to stick out – cables, brakes – is being concealed. Frame material continues to evolve, too, with lighter and stronger carbon fibre hitting the market all the time; in fact, that's a key reason why aerodynamic road bikes have taken off. In the past, adding the extra carbon required for that teardrop shape increased weight, so was only deemed beneficial for time trials where a lack of drafting and peloton meant aerodynamics were deemed more important than for a traditional road stage. Now, advances in material technology has seen lighter and stiffer carbon flood the market, meaning road bikes can now enjoy the

▽ Miguel Indurain
of Spain and team
Banesto is pursued
by Luc Leblanc on
Stage 16 of the Tour
de France between
Valreas and
L'Alpe d'Huez

aerodynamic advantage once reserved for TTs. See the 'Carbon fibre in 2016' box (page 96) for further detail on carbon fibre and its use in the peloton.

It's a far cry from when Maurice Garin won the first Tour de France in 1903, covering the six-stage 2,428km race in just over 94 hours, the spirited Frenchman riding to victory on a bike constructed from heavy steel. Those early bikes weighed over 16kg – twice that of today's svelte models. As the years rolled by, steel continued to dominate the Tour – though lighter, stronger tubing from, most notably, Reynolds and Columbus saw bike weight drop to around the 8–10kg mark – until Spain's Miguel Indurain won the fourth of his five Tour titles in 1994. Indurain's victory on a Pinarello-badged bike signalled the last time a steel bike won the Tour.

1999 was the first time a full carbon bike won the Tour, Lance Armstrong riding the Trek 5500 to the first of seven titles that were subsequently wiped from the record books. At the time, Trek made much of how it was the first time a carbon bike had been ridden from start to finish at the Tour. But it wasn't the first time carbon had infiltrated the Tour.

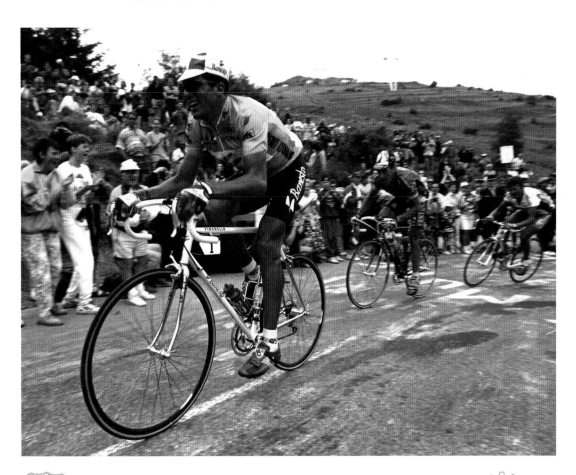

# Carbon fibre in 2016

○ French bicycle manufacturer

Look is a regular on the Tour, most recently providing the bikes for French team Bretagne-Séché Environnement at the 2015 Tour. Here, Look general manager Jean-Claude Chrétien, who's primarily based at their Tunisian manufacturing plant, explains the difference between the carbon used on their bikes:

'We use carbon fibre that has been impregnated with an epoxy resin, which adds strength and structure to the carbon fibres during the manufacturing process. Carbonisation takes place between 1,000–1,050°C and results in a fibre that's 90 per cent carbon and 10 per cent oxygen. This is what we term high resistance (HR) and is characterised by a slightly less rigid feel, so is good for components that might need a touch more flex.

'If you crank the furnace up to 1,500°C, each fibre will contain 99 per cent carbon and just 1 per cent oxygen. This is known as high modulus (HM; modulus means tensile strength) and is very rigid, so good for power transfer but is brittle and can break easily if hit side on.

'As a matter of comparison, HR breaks at 24 tons of pressure, Intermediate Modulus (IM) 30 tons and HM 40 tons, but HR and IM can elongate by 2.5 per cent before breaking, unlike HM which is 1.5 per cent. That's why we use a mix of the three different fibres in our top-end 795.

'Our R&D department decide on which fibre goes where on the bike. They also decide on resin content. This can be up to 40 per cent. When you're using high strength fibre, you need more resin because it's more difficult to impregnate.'

'I made the first carbon frame back in 1982,' says Jean-Marc Gueugneaud, who now works for French carbon bike manufacturers Time, who are based near Lyon. 'I was working at Mercier just south-west of here. We produced metallic frames and nearly won the Tour, twice finishing second with Raymond Poulidor and Joop Zoetemelk. While there, a colleague asked for a solution to his prototype and I offered my expertise. I made the first carbon bike on a jig and joined it with lugs.'

Gueugneaud was surprised by the results, went freelance and continued to develop the technology. At the same time, the French Aerospace Company TVT (Technique du Verre Tissé) were looking to make their presence felt in the world of cycling and recruited Gueugneaud to their ranks where he helped them make the first carbon frame and fork combination. Then, at a trade show in Paris, his good friend Alain Decroix asked him if he'd provide a bike for Bernard Hinault, for whom Decroix worked as a mechanic.

'Of course, I said yes,' he says. 'Hinault rode it during the winter of '85–'86. He liked the bike and, in February '86, rode it during the first stage of the Tour de Méditerranéean. I didn't even know he was going to and it was always difficult to ask Bernard a question! He then had a few bad comments but I was confident in the frame and it turned out the problems were with the fork.'

That night, the new carbon fork was replaced by a steel one. Hinault was delighted with the outcome, though race victory went to his La Vie Claire teammate Jean-François Bernard. The Badger, though, had seen enough to convince him that his team should ride the bikes at that year's Tour de France.

'That was a confusing one,' says Gueugneaud. 'La Vie Claire was sponsored by Look. Both were owned by Bernard Tapie. Hinault was a legend and his word goes so, come the Tour, the team is riding TVT frames with Look and Reynolds tubing branding.' So that iconic image of LeMond and Hinault, hand in hand as they approach the finish line of the 1986 stage in Alpe d'Huez, insincerity reverberating from every pedal stroke, is actually aboard Jean-Marc's handiwork.

'We also gave Pedro Delgado a bike for the 1988 Tour and he got into trouble with Pinarello and Columbus [steel tubing]. But he was in yellow and told everyone he'd win the race on this bike. Stage after stage, more and more Columbus stickers plastered the frame. It must have weighed him down! Delgado won and it was quite funny. At the start of the season, TVT only sold blue bikes. Pedro won on a red TVT [Pinarello] so by the end of that race, everyone unknowingly wanted a red TVT!'

Branding bikes and components not from the team's bike sponsor is nothing new, and like the instances of dopers being struck from the record books it makes charting the evolution of frame design a labyrinth. What's clear, though, is that every single team in the WorldTour now uses carbon bicycles. And that's set to stay, according to industry experts.

'I can't see carbon being threatened in the future,' says Gerard Vroomen, formerly of Cervélo. 'Carbon will continue to be developed, though you might also have high-performance stuff ranging from nanotechnology to graphene. We'll see what makes it big in cycling.'

For now, the UCI's minimum weight limit of 6.8kg means aerodynamics will continue to dominate the focus of the bike industry, though that could revert back to their historic focus on weight if the UCI lowers that mark. Whether that would mean aerodynamics, which requires more tubing than is traditional for that airfoil shape, would be sacrificed for weight losses remains to be seen.

For now, the riders at the Tour employ a time-trial bike for time trials, and then either a road or aero road bike for the road stages, depending on the profile of the course (see the 'Which bike?' box on page 100). Lighter, more traditional road bikes like the Specialized Tarmac used by Nibali and Contador tend to dominate the hills but ultimately it's down to the rider. And professional cyclists are a pernickety lot.

'We have three to choose from,' says Lotto-Soudal's Greg Henderson. 'We have the Ridley Noah SL aero road bike, which is typically the sprint bike – it's a little heavier and a little stiffer because there's more carbon around the bottom bracket for extra power. We have the Helium SL, which is a super lightweight frame that you can get right down to 6.8kg and even under. Then there's the Phoenix SL, which is

 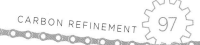

more of a long wheelbase [measurement between wheel axles; longer equals greater comfort, shorter is better for handling] and one the boys use more for the Classics.'

'Myself, I use the Noah,' he adds. 'I'm really pedantic about my seat height. Really pedantic about my position. I can feel 1mm change on seat height. And it just feels like a better position on the Noah SL. However, I've put it on its own special diet for big races, using all sorts of little tricks, like using titanium bolt kits, to shave weight off so it can get as close as possible to the minimum weight of 6.8kg. So I don't have to ride the Helium and still have it at a good weight.'

Henderson describes himself as a micro-adjuster, a term coined by Team Sky physio-therapist Phil Burt for riders who feel like they make big gains from the tiniest of tweaks. 'That's certainly true for me, especially when it comes to wheel selection,' he says. 'I was always taught at my time with Team Sky and HTC that rotational weight is worth twice that of stacking weight.' In other words, a rotational weight creates twice the downward force as the weight on a non-moving object, like a frame.

# THE DEEP-RIM REVOLUTION

Wheel selection used to be a pretty straight-forward affair, the rider choosing between tubulars and clinchers (tubulars stick to the tyre so you can inflate to greater pressures, which could equate to more speed; clinchers are the inner tube-and-tyre combo and can't be inflated as high but are easier to maintain) and how many spokes they wanted. Then along came American Steve Hed who helped to reinvent the sector. 'Many of my triathlon friends were competing at Ironman Hawaii, including my wife Annie,' Hed told me before he sadly passed

## Which bike?

○ Specialized's Chris Yu is an aerodynamicist, so knows a thing or two about carving through the path of least resistance. Here, he explains the tests he's undertaken to ascertain when to use the Tarmac road bike, Venge aero road bike and Shiv time-trial bike...

'There are a few comparisons we've undertaken,' says Yu. 'With no rider on-board, we've compared the 'typical' road bike, featuring traditional tube shaping, shallow-rimmed wheels and round handlebars, similar to our Tarmac SL4 (prior to the current Tarmac which actually has some subtle aero shaping to it), to the latest-generation aero system, namely the Venge ViAS including aerodynamic frame and fork, fully integrated cockpit and brakes, and deep-section wheels. In this case, we've found that the Venge ViAS is about 120 seconds faster over 40km than the traditional road bike.

'We've also compared the Venge ViAS to our Shiv time-trial bike, which also rolled on deep-section wheels. This was in the wind tunnel and without a rider. We discovered that both bikes were aerodynamically very similar. Where things really differ arises from a rider on-board as the aerobars allow the rider to nestle down into a more aerodynamic, slipstreamed position.'

Ultimately, the lightweight Tarmac comes into its own when the course profile features many hills; the Venge can handle the hills but performs at its peak in flatter road stages; and the Shiv is for out-and-out time trials.

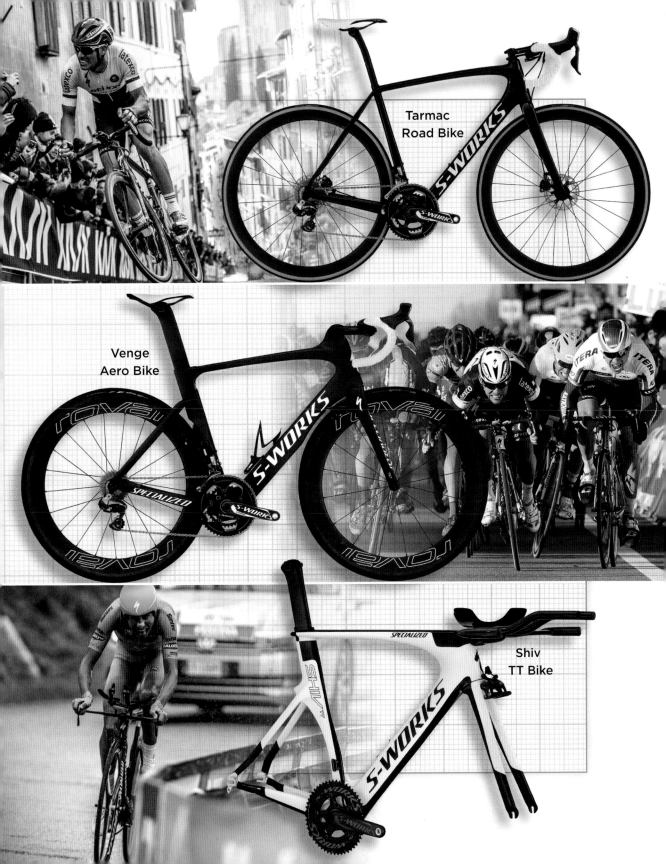

Tarmac
Road Bike

Venge
Aero Bike

Shiv
TT Bike

away at the end of 2014. 'Because of the strong winds in Kona, disc wheels are banned. So I went back to the drawing board and came up with the Hed CX, the first deep-section rim.'

Hed's deep-section rims worked, and you only need to glance at the peloton and you'll see how they proliferate through the pro ranks, providing drag savings that result in more speed. As for disc wheels, like in the Ironman Hawaii they're banned in the peloton. UCI rules state that: 'For mass competitions on the road … wheels shall have at least 12 spokes'. The maximum extension of the wheel rim for these mass-start stages is 65mm.

In the peloton there is choppy, unpredictable air and lots of handling issues just keeping upright alongside 200 other riders, meaning it's not possible to use full disc wheels, which handle less sensitively and are very wobbly in high winds. But, disc wheels *are* allowed in time trials, where riders set off individually one or two minutes apart, so teams can throw their full aerodynamic weight behind the team, and disc wheels and tri-spokes (front wheel with just three spokes) are the norm.

'I'll always run rear disc wheel in a time trial,' says Movistar's time-trialling specialist Alex Dowsett. 'As for the front, that's down to the course profile and weather. The wind, in particular, has a role to play and dictates whether I go for a 40mm-deep rim or 80mm. The wind doesn't really affect the rear but it does the front because of handling.'

Dowsett recalls when he time-trialled for Trek-Livestrong at the 2010 Tour of the Gila and ran a 60mm upfront and disc wheel at the rear. His main rivals, Tom Danielson and Levi Leipheimer, went for 80mm-deep wheels front and rear. All three competitors chose the wrong combination. 'It turned out that horrendous crosswinds were sweeping over the course and the bike was a nightmare to handle. We were all beaten by my teammate of the time, Jesse Sergent, who ran a disc in the rear but a climbing wheel upfront. It had no rim depth at all but he destroyed everyone because he didn't have to fight his bike.'

Balancing aerodynamics with handling is how Enve wheels have grown into one of the most well-respected wheel manufacturers on the circuit. They're used by Team Dimension Data but are cast over by envious eyes. 'I've used Campagnolo's Bora for a few years now and they're cracking wheels,' says Henderson, 'but I know there's some amazing technology out there now, specifically from Zipp and Enve.' Wheel manufacturers pay teams to use their wheels, so each rider must use the team's sponsored wheels.

While Campagnolo's bike heritage stretches back to 1933, Enve is a relatively young company, founded by cousins Brett and Taylor Satterthwaite in 2007 in Utah, America. In 2011 they hooked up with aerodynamicist Simon Smart and began rolling out their road range with one key feature: stability.

'There were some great wheels out there by people like Zipp and Hed but, in my opinion, they were being let down by handling,' explains Smart. 'Loads of

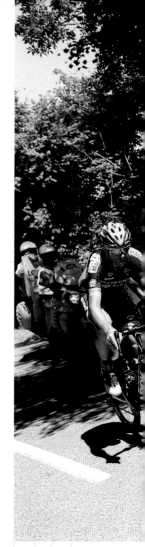

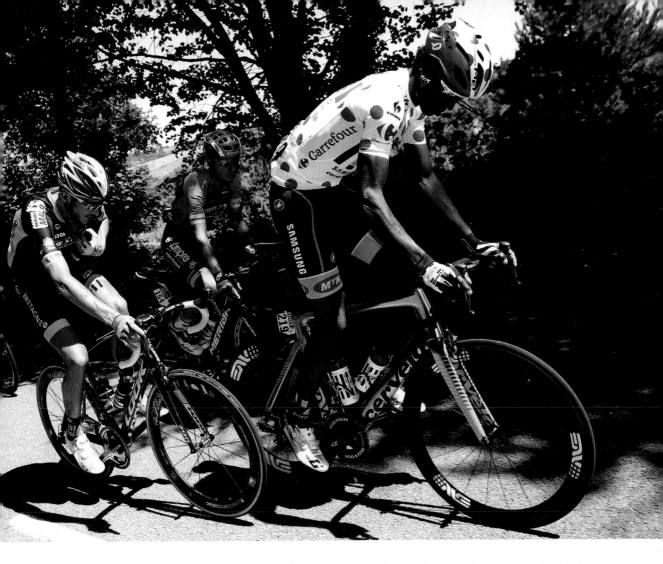

△ Daniel
Teklehaimanot of
Eritrea and MTN-
Qhubeka competes
during stage seven
of the 2015 Tour de
France, between
Livarot and Fougeres

wheel manufacturers were making huge claims about performance in the wind-tunnel, but that wasn't reflected out on the road. And the reason? Because they were testing wheels in isolation. As soon as they were slotted into the frames, they behaved completely differently.

'Key to maintaining stability of a wheel is to reduce or delay the separation of airflow on the rims,' Smart continues. 'That makes them more predictable, especially on the front wheel, which you have to handle. We looked at steering torque [when steering begins to veer left or right], which is generated in a crosswind. We had two philosophies: to either reduce torque or to go with it but ensuring the wheel behaves in a predictable manner.'

Smart and Enve chose the latter, remedying the problem by not only manipulating rim shapes, but also by making the rear wheel deeper to reduce drag where stability's less of an issue. They achieved this by making the front wheel rim wider and shallower (26mm wide, 85mm deep, for example) compared to the rear wheel, which measured 24mm and 95mm, respectively. This was for time trials.

Bike manufacturers are seemingly paying more attention than ever before to stability, with Zipp's bulbous Firecrest 808 wheels feeling similar in crosswinds to a much-shallower rim. Still, despite this wheel revolution, the issue of handling and stability was very much brought into focus in 2014 with a series of high-profile crashes. Irony poured from the skies at the Tour de France as raw, lush Yorkshire remained dry, while France drowned in a daily deluge. The riders had to wait until the first rest day before the rain subsided. By then, the stage penned 'the battlefield' (stage five between Ypres and Arenberg Porte de Hainaut) had sent Chris Froome's chances of retaining the title packing into one of Sky's Jaguars after he'd crashed three times in 24 hours.

Froome wasn't the only one. Ag2r's Sébastien Minard skidded near a round-about, losing his bike from beneath him; Giant-Shimano's Marcel Kittel did the same around a corner, breaking his cleats. With 70km to go, as the peloton split as

▽ Steven Kruijswijk (L) sits on the ground after a big crash during the 189.5km fifth stage of the 102nd edition of the Tour de France cycling race on July 8, 2015, between Arras and Amiens

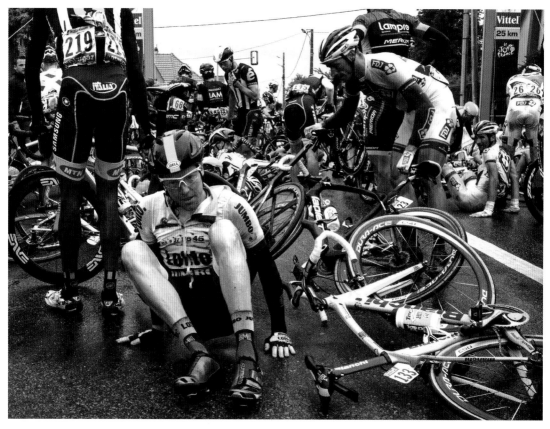

it swept around a giant roundabout, there were crashes on both sides of the road, including Movistar's Alejandro Valverde and BMC Racing's Tejay van Garderen.

The rain, crosswinds and tension of the early stages of the 2014 Tour had conspired to create absolute carnage. While the cobbles and weather took their toll, some critics blamed the deep rims and the subsequent uncertain, choppy airflow of riding in a peloton. Paul Lew, director of technology and innovation at Reynolds Wheels, plays down those concerns and argues the opposite.

'The UCI has set a maximum depth of 65mm rims for mass-start races to ensure that a wheel will not handle adversely in high-wind conditions,' he says. 'While the intention of the regulation is understandable, the result limits innovation. Let me explain how. We use Reynolds's DET technology (dispersive effect termination), which has changed the way wind reacts to a deep-section wheel. For instance, our 72mm-deep aero wheel has a steering torque similar to our Assault/Forty-Six, which has a depth of 46mm, so in high wind conditions the 72 Aero will generate a similar risk to the rider as a 46mm wheel, so why not allow this wheel for mass start competition?'

Whether the Tour rider would choose to select a 72mm rim remains to be seen. Despite advances in carbon-fibre technology and greater handleability in the wind, a shallower-rimmed wheel, like the 46mm example, is always going to be lighter than one that's loaded with an extra-deep section of carbon. And to the very best riders in the peloton, that's vital.

'If the course profile is lumpy and twisting left and right, I want it as light as possible so that it'll respond to acceleration faster than a big, heavy deep-section wheel,' says Greg Henderson. 'For me, weight is one of the major factors of wheel selection.'

# ACCELERATION CONSIDERATIONS

Physics dictates that the rotating-weight penalty (heavier wheels) only really affects acceleration, so for many riders on a flat stage, deeper rims should be the norm. However, for a sprinter like Henderson, where a millisecond of indecision could be the difference between success and disappointment, weight is crucial.

'I look at it like a percentage of body weight,' explains Henderson. 'The big sprinters like Andre Greipel and Marcel Kittel, who are around 85–90kg, they have a lot more power at their disposal than guys like myself who weigh between 69kg and 70kg. When you look at overall weight of me, frame and wheel compared to Kittel, the wheel's a higher weight percentage and that needs to be powered up and accelerated. It's the same with climbers who might weigh near 50kg. They have to be super-pernickety when it comes to wheel selection. Lighter is often better.'

At the 2014 Tour, Nibali often chose the Corima 32mm-deep Viva S hoops that weigh a meagre 1,190g for the pair. As the gradient rises and the sprinter sprints,

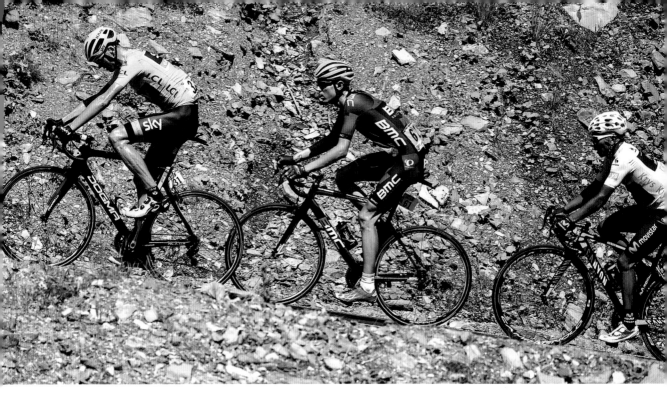

shallower rims are often better. 'Everyday each rider makes a wheel decision and asks the mechanic to put it on their bike for the next day,' says über-climber Bauke Mollema of Trek-Segafredo. 'I always ride 50mm-deep wheels from Bontrager on flat stages but, for the climbs, I drop to 30mm. It's all a balance of weight and aero-dynamics but definitely lighter is better for me when climbing.'

And that's all down to inertia. Inertia is based on the principle that mass away from the centre of rotation is harder to rotate than when close to the centre of rotation. In cycling, of course, the centre is the hub and the outer rotation is the rim. Newton's Second Law says that the sum of all forces is the same as inertia multiplied by the angle of acceleration. So if inertia is high, it'll require greater force to move.

'Consider a figure skater rotating on the spot with her arms spread out,' says Marco Arkesteijn, sport and exercise scientist at Aberystwyth University. 'She rotates around the mid-point of the body – the part that's stationary. This is her centre of rotation. She increases her rotation velocity by tucking her hands into her body. What she's doing is decreasing the mass away from the centre of rotation, which lowers the inertia. As her momentum is constant, it follows from Newton's Second Law that her angular acceleration increases and so her velocity increases.'

So that's why lower weight at the rim equals faster accelerations, and probably has you questioning why the professionals don't use smaller wheels, like 650c wheels (often used by female riders) over the 700c standard. Tests by Cervélo showed 650c wheels created 8–12 per cent less drag than 700c versions, though

△ Chris Froome, Tejay Van Garderen and Nairo Quintana wisely all choose lighter shallower rims on the hills

rolling resistance increases because of the smaller wheel; in other words, the 650c wheel has to revolve more times than the 700c wheel to achieve the same speed.

Back to our skater's analogy and the issue of rim weight on acceleration, you can see the advantage of a light rim when a puncheur like Philippe Gilbert sprints up a short climb. Mavic's Product Manager Maxime Brunand rolled out an experiment that highlighted this concept further. She added 50g to two sets of wheels – one at the rim, one at the hub – and had a rider power up to 500 watts on a 10 per cent gradient and saw how long it took them to reach 20km/h.

'We discovered that the wheel with added rim weight took five times longer to reach 20km/h than when that weight was added on that rim on the flat,' she says. 'At the hub, it took just four times as long to reach its horizontal speed. Essentially, on hills, inertia becomes more important.'

Brunand and her team also showed there was no significant difference between added rim or hub weight on reaching 36km/h on the flat at 500 watts. However, the French team also observed that because greater kinetic energy was required to accelerate the rim-based weight wheel up to speed, 'it was easier to maintain speed'. Which very much conforms to the idea of deep (heavier) rims for maintaining and increasing momentum.

## Carrying the bikes

○ The Tour de France teams have two team cars that follow the race. Inside the car is usually a *directeur sportif* (DS), who'll direct rider strategy on the fly as well as drive the car, and a mechanic, who'll sit on a back seat and feed water bottles and food to the DS, who'll then pass these on to the domestique.

Each of the team's nine riders is allocated one spare bike per car. 'Each car can take up to nine bikes,' says Trek-Segafredo mechanic Mauro Abobati. 'However, because of space restrictions, only four of the bikes will be clamped into place with wheels on. Those are on the outer edges of the roof and are more easily accessed for the most important riders. This could be a rider who's in contention for general classification or a rider who's vital for a specific stage, like a sprinter. The remaining five bikes are fixed into place but their wheels are in the boot.'

If an important rider – say the GC contender – crashes and the team cars can't reach him swiftly, often a teammate (a domestique) will sacrifice their bike. The car will then deposit a spare bike to the 'bikeless rider', pick up the crashed bike and accelerate up to the GC rider. The GC rider will then take delivery of his spare bike – the domestique's bike might have different tubing lengths, for example. At this point, the mechanic will look to repair the GC contender's original bike, just in case he needs it later in the stage. Comprende?!

 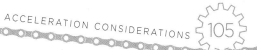

# TYRE WIDTH

You can't discuss the Tour and wheel selection without mentioning the *service des courses*. This is a neutral mechanical service that Mavic has provided at one-day Classics and multi-stage races for over 40 years. In 1972, a team manager's car broke down while following the Critérium du Dauphiné. Mavic's chairman at the time, Bruno Gormand, lent his own car to the manager and the idea was born. A year later, Mavic's neutral service appeared officially for the first time at Paris–Nice and has been supporting riders in breakaways and in the peloton ever since.

'In 2014 we covered 89 events, across all forms. That's professional, amateur, sportives and mountain bike,' says Michel Lethenet, Mavic's global PR manager. 'The Tour is obviously very important but the most debilitating is Paris–Roubaix where we have 17 people involved. That's on top of four cars, four motorbikes, one lorry and 120 pairs of wheels. Though we still have more people and vehicles involved at the Tour, it's just as tiring.'

Many of those wheels would have featured tyres of around 25mm in width. This is a recent advancement as thinner was always thought to be better – 23mm wide used to be the norm, though 19mm wasn't unheard of – the reason being that the thinner the contact with the ground, the less rolling resistance, plus the thinner the tyre, the lighter it was. But an increasing number of manufacturers are creating wider tyres because of a collective about-turn on what makes a fast tyre.

'At the same pressure, a 25mm tyre is 7 per cent faster than a 22mm,' says Christian Wurmbaeck, product manager at Continental Tyres. 'It started in 2013. First, teams like BMC switched to 25mm. Before it was just 19 and 22mm. Now nearly all teams use 25mm wheels. That's predominantly down to the improvement in aerodynamics.'

The theory goes that a 25mm-wide tubular tyre fits better onto a wheel than a thinner tyre. That has the effect of smoothing out airflow between the wheel and tyre, rather than creating a choppy effect if the tyre's too thin. Rolling resistance is purportedly no more, too, due to something called tyre deflection. At the same tyre pressure, a wide and narrow tyre has the same contact area as a thinner tyre because while the wide tyre is flattened over its width, the narrower tyre flattens over its length. They're also more comfortable than thinner tyres because of the greater volume of air between you and the road.

That thickness rises at cobbled stages, seen at both the 2014 and 2015 Tours, where teams migrate to 27mm or 28mm thick tyres and lower tyre pressures to cope with the jagged terrain.

'Tyres are clearly very important and have a huge impact on how you ride, including things like handling,' says Wurmbaeck. 'It's the whole tyre construction, from the construction of the tread to whether you use puncture-resistance layers like Vectran, which is super-stiff but if you put too much material in it, the tyre

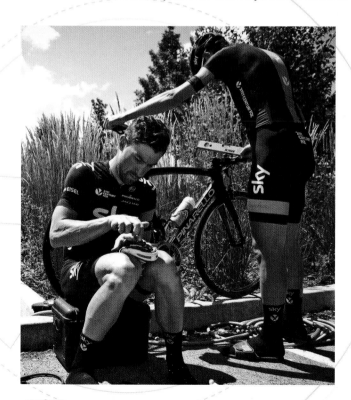

just feels slow. The inner tube, too – do you use butyl rubber or Latex? Each rides slightly differently.'

Tyre design and manufacture, just like the frames and wheels, continues to evolve. Science is turning concepts taken as gospel, like the thickness of a tyre, on their head, but where is this evolution heading in the future? Before he passed away, Steve Hed told me, 'The answer to the question depends who you ask. For the most part, frame designers say frames, wheel designers say wheels, tyre designers say tyres. I say all three. The interaction between frame, wheel and tyre is one of the significant areas of focus for aerodynamic improvement. I estimate that another 30 per cent of aerodynamic efficiency can be realised by investigating this interaction. It's easy to see in aerodynamic analysis that the drag from the integration of the front wheel and fork is nearly equal to the drag of the wheel as a stand-alone component, but not very much work has been done to improve the fork-frame-to-wheel interaction. Collaboration between frame and wheel companies will undoubtedly begin to take on a more important role. In the future I see a more integrated performance-based approach.'

The industry tends to agree with Hed. 'We're in constant dialogue with frame manufacturers and that can only be a good thing for integration and improved aerodynamics,' adds Reynolds's Paul Lew. 'There's more conversation now between wheel and frame manufacturers than there ever has been in my 25 years in the industry.'

Clearly there'll be hurdles to innovation, specifically from the UCI's remit to make sure machine doesn't eclipse man in importance. As Hed and Lew said, frame and wheel makers will have to work more closely together than ever before, suggesting bike manufacturers like Trek and Specialized, who also have the financial clout to create their own wheels – Bontrager and Roval, respectively – may well gain a competitive advantage over their more piecemeal rivals. Wherever the future lies, you can guarantee that it'll be very, very fast, and as you'll discover next, it will be ably supported by further drag savings in the form of clothing, helmets and components.

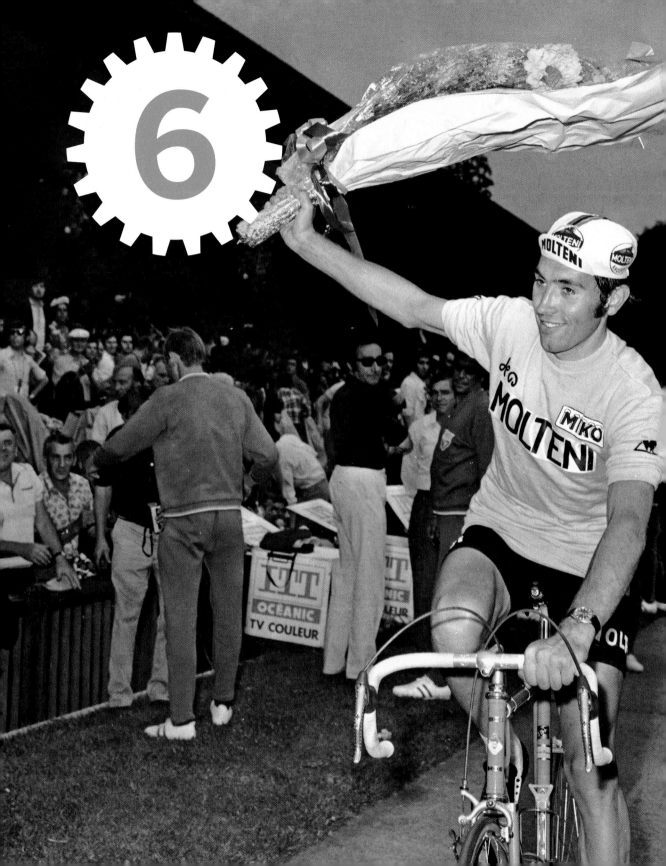

# SUPPLEMENTING SPEED
## CLOTHING, HELMETS AND SADDLES

**Mario Cipollini was once quoted** as saying, 'If I wasn't a professional bike rider, I'd be a porn star.' 'Cipo' was never short of confidence, but had form to back up the rhetoric, the Italian sprinter winning 191 times, including 12 stages of the Tour de France, in 16 years from 1989 to 2005 (though he briefly returned in 2008 with Rock Racing). Over the course of 'Super' Mario's professional career, he also courted controversy, becoming famous for his extravagant attire, including custom-made skinsuits patterned in zebra, tiger and, one for the happy hardcore, techno symbols. Cipollini's decorative wardrobe captured the headlines and was a world away from the traditional woolen outfits of years gone by.

Wool used to dominate the professional cyclist's wardrobe, the orange Molteni-sponsored jersey of Eddy Merckx a classic of the genre. Wool moved moisture away from the skin more proficiently than cotton and absorbed perspiration better. The problem was, it offered little cooling, so you heated up rapidly, leaving the woollen top a soaked mess. That affected the garment's shape (and smell), creating a baggy sack. Wool's dominance on the professional cyclist's catwalk lasted until the 1980s when the industry finally awoke to the benefits of not only polyester but also polyester combined with elastic, namely Lycra. Polyester transferred sweat to the open air with improved efficiency and, as Cipollini showed, could be printed with far more vivid colours and patterns than wool. But it's the tight fit that offered riders the greatest benefits – and that's once again down to aerodynamics.

◁ Eddy Merckx celebrates his fourth consecutive win in the Tour de France, 1972, adorned in his famous Molteni woolen jersey

## Secret Squirrel Club

○ After the 2004 Athens Olympics, where GB won two cycling medals, performance director Dave Brailsford and Chris Boardman had one of their regular meetings in a Starbucks coffee shop. Despite Sir Bradley Wiggins' and Chris Hoy's success, GB retained the reputation as King of the Qualifiers and, as Boardman says, were still considered shite when it mattered.

'We wanted to lose that image, obviously,' Boardman explains. 'We discussed it and we felt there was a huge number of smaller developments that could make you go quicker. So I was officially appointed Head of Stuff. It ended up Marginal Gains but really it was Head of Stuff.' This signalled the creation of the Secret Squirrel Club, a select group that included Brailsford, Boardman and a band of sports scientists looking for cutting-edge advancements.

'I spent loads of time going around the world and talking to manufacturers,' adds Boardman. 'Our line was performance first and then work out if we had enough funding. Thankfully the Lottery put us in a privileged position because we didn't have to satiate commercial demands. It was all about performance.'

British Cycling began spending more and more time in the wind tunnel, primarily at Southampton University, and by the London Olympics in 2012 they'd produced 28 major projects. These included the Datarider, a black-box recorder the size of a matchbox that sat beneath the saddle and recorded performance measurements.

'All the big ideas came from the non-biking industry. We visited the military, F1, academia, aviation… When we first went to McLaren, we discovered they knew nothing about cycling. They always asked: why do you do that? And we replied, we don't know. You suddenly realise how restricted by tradition you are. For example, if I say to a rider, do you use 39cm bars? They might say yes. What about 27s? No? Why not? What is your rationale for not doing that? A mix of ignorance and expertise is the ideal marriage for breaking boundaries.'

Boardman and Brailsford are no longer with the Secret Squirrels, though it survives to this day, continuing the progressive work of their high-profile former custodians.

'Around 80 per cent of the frontal area facing the air is the rider,' says Chris Boardman, who became synonymous with innovation and aerodynamics, first as a rider and then as part of British Cycling's so called Secret Squirrel Club (see above). 'Anything you can do to reduce that figure helps you go faster, and that's why clothing's so important.'

Boardman recalls racing a domestic event in England back in the 1980s. Ever the innovator, Boardman wore a tight-fitting suit that resembled a leotard, much to the ridicule of his competitors. 'Then I pissed them off and won it,' he says. 'Nowadays you'd be mocked if you didn't wear a skinsuit during a time trial.'

# TIME-TRIALLING CATWALK

The time trial is the discipline that's historically attracted the biggest aerodynamic developments. In fact, so important is time-trialling to some cyclists' chances of winning the Tour de France that Bradley Wiggins' 2012 triumph was attributed to a time-trial friendly route. Wiggins, of course, further highlighted his time-trialling pedigree in June 2015 when he broke the one-hour world record.

Wiggins bettered his English compatriot Alex Dowsett's time, who races for Spanish team Movistar. In the build-up to his record-breaking attempt, Dowsett spent hours in the Formula One wind tunnel at Brackley, England, and on the track testing skin suits made by Scottish manufacturer Endura, who are kit suppliers to Movistar. 'We made 57 versions of the Aero Speedsuit featuring 30 different fabrics,' explains Endura brand manager Ian Young. 'We also spent more than 24 hours in the wind tunnel to create a suit that recorded the lowest drag.'

Not all of those 24 hours were ridden by Alex, of course – he has road races to compete in – so Endura employed a typical trick of the bike clothing industry and tested developments on an employee who has similar dimensions to Dowsett. Dowsett's Aero Speedsuit was a joint venture between Endura and the man behind Enve wheels and the Scott Plasma bike, aerodynamicist Simon Smart.

'We've been developing clothing for about five years now for time-triallists,' explains Smart. 'But everything was bespoke and we couldn't increase volume of sales without a partner, so we hooked up with Endura who almost had the opposite

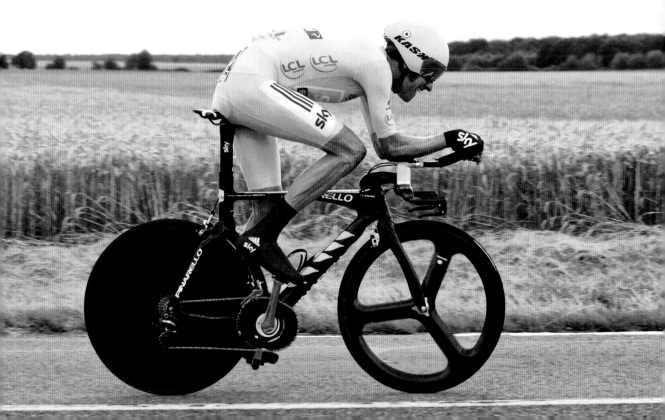

problem. They had the clothing facilities but didn't have the aerodynamic know-how.'

Endura are understandably reluctant to reveal too much about the composition of Dowsett's speedsuit – though educated opinion suggests a polyester weave was at its heart – but Young does reveal, 'The suit employed three different fabrics. There were minimal seams – the body panel is all one piece – and it's designed to sustain an aerodynamic position. You also probably noticed the zip on the back, which was mainly there for improved fit, comfort and making it easier to slip on and off.'

It's not all about the physical advantage – the right suit can gain you a psychological edge, too. 'For the 2014 Commonwealth Games time trial, Endura produced three different suits for me,' says Dowsett. 'I remember driving up to their factory in Scotland to pick them up. We'd tested them in the wind tunnel and they were faster than my existing kit, but then they noticed the smallest wrinkle on the shoulders. As far as I was concerned it was fine, but they worked through the night to build me a new suit, taking 15mm off the shoulders.

'Come the race I'm in the warm-up tent and Steve Cummings is on the turbo trainer. I pulled out my new suit. He looked at his, looked at mine, and said the suit looked different and fast. I said, "Yeah, doesn't get any quicker than this, I'm afraid". Then I pulled out these overshoes that Endura had made me and he just went, "For fuck's sake, Alex". I remember thinking right there that I'd beaten him before I'd turned a pedal stroke.'

Dowsett beat Cummings by over 1:30 minutes. In fact, over the 40km loop around the streets of Glasgow, Dowsett beat everyone, including Australia's Rohan Dennis to the gold medal by less than 10 seconds. 'I raced for nearly 50 minutes [47 minutes, 41 seconds] and won by such a small margin that the new speedsuit could have been the difference between gold and silver,' he says. 'Clothing choice really matters.'

It's a sentiment echoed by arguably the era's greatest cyclist – Alberto Contador. At stage 10 of the 2014 Vuelta, Contador finished 39 seconds behind the day's winner, Tony Martin of Omega Pharma-QuickStep. The 36.7km time trial weaved its way through the tricky backstreets of Real Monasterio de Santa Maria de Veruela before ascending over hills that include a category-two climb (more on hill categorisation in Chapter 8). Contador, a good time-triallist but no Tony Martin, flew around the course, beating traditionally stronger time-triallists like Chris Froome to ride into the race's red jersey. It was a lead he never relinquished en route to his sixth major victory.

That day, the world saw a sinewy, tanned Contador once again prove he's one of the world's most versatile riders. Steve Smith, brand manager at Sportful who supply kit to Tinkoff Sport, saw something different. 'That was the culmination of a project that cost around €400,000,' says Smith. 'We made Contador a custom-made skinsuit … and clearly it was worth it.'

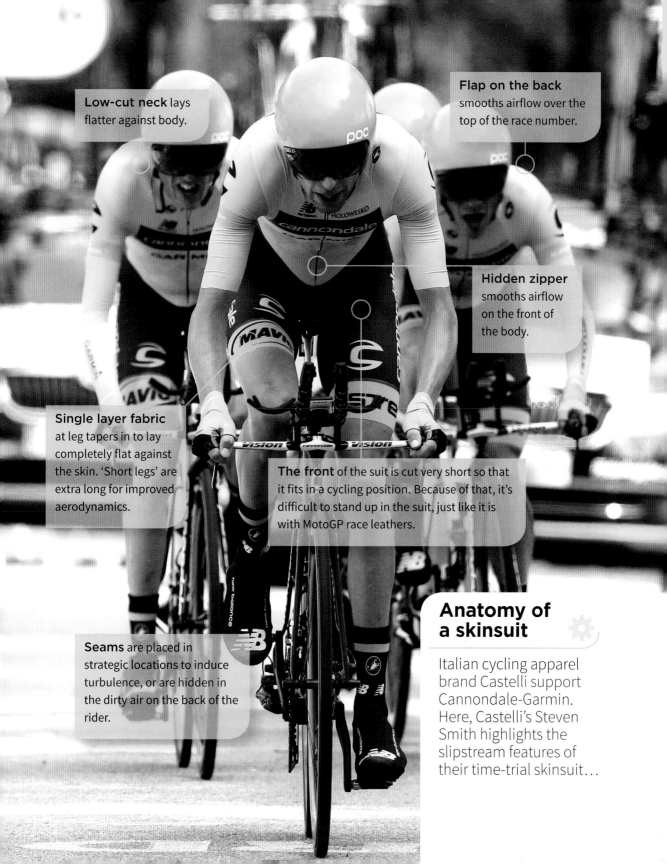

**Low-cut neck** lays flatter against body.

**Flap on the back** smooths airflow over the top of the race number.

**Hidden zipper** smooths airflow on the front of the body.

**Single layer fabric** at leg tapers in to lay completely flat against the skin. 'Short legs' are extra long for improved aerodynamics.

**The front** of the suit is cut very short so that it fits in a cycling position. Because of that, it's difficult to stand up in the suit, just like it is with MotoGP race leathers.

**Seams** are placed in strategic locations to induce turbulence, or are hidden in the dirty air on the back of the rider.

## Anatomy of a skinsuit

Italian cycling apparel brand Castelli support Cannondale-Garmin. Here, Castelli's Steven Smith highlights the slipstream features of their time-trial skinsuit…

# BESPOKE SPEED

▷ Alberto Contador of Spain riding for Tinkoff-Saxo, competing in the individual time trial in stage one of the 2015 Tour de France

The long process of dressing a legend began at the start of 2014 when Sportful's aerodynamics team analysed Contador's time-trial position through their computational fluid dynamics software to create a virtual, on-screen Contador. 'We monitored the motion of his body as it travels through the air,' says Smith. 'Alberto's fairly broad in the shoulders and narrow at the waist, so from that and the data, we could work out the ideal seam placement and fabric for Alberto.'

With data in the bag, Sportful set about creating Contador's custom-made suit. Probed on the processes and fabrics required, Smith says he can't give away the brand's secrets. More intellectual property. What we do know is that this €400,000 investment isn't the norm. In general, Sportful don't make custom-made kit for the professionals; instead they use regular and long cuts that cover 95 per cent of the professionals 'because they're tall and skinny'. 'If Alberto wants a further 2cm off the waist of a standard kit, we'll do that for him,' says Smith. 'If it's a neo-pro who hasn't earned his stripes yet, we might just tell them to pedal a little bit harder!'

David Martin, of the Australian Institute of Sport (AIS) and Orica GreenEdge, was more candid about the work his team has been undertaking. 'It's called Project Aerotwin,' says Martin. 'Basically, it involves a wind-tunnel and mannequins.' But these are no ordinary mannequins. The AIS designed them to conform to the morphology of individual riders, and they are mobile and limber enough to pedal in the same style as a professional.

'The aim is that every rider has their body dimensions mapped by a scanner, which sends the data through a computer before a separate machine creates the mannequin. 'It's not quite there yet but we'd have a Simon Gerrans mannequin, a Michael Matthews mannequin …'

Currently, they're working with just the one mobile mannequin and shaping its dimensions to suit the specific statistics of the respective rider. But with further funding, a slightly eerie peloton will inhabit the AIS.

'The idea is to play around with different types of fabrics and textures and skinsuits on the mannequin,' Martin explains. 'Like one-off bespoke suits, the question changes from "what's the best skinsuit" to "what's the best skinsuit for you?" The difference is we can really work on the detail while the riders are off racing thanks to the mannequins.'

Each mannequin is designed to be as realistic as possible, so you can tilt its moving parts in the same planes of movement as a human being. And the researchers can play around with yaw angles so that the wind isn't always coming directly onto the riders; it'll come from maybe across the shoulder, again to mimic real life.

'We can then see what a skinsuit looks like that's really slippery in the air. There are a couple of things you can play with. You can keep the fabric smooth to carve through the air. Or you can rough up the fabric, maybe putting dimples on

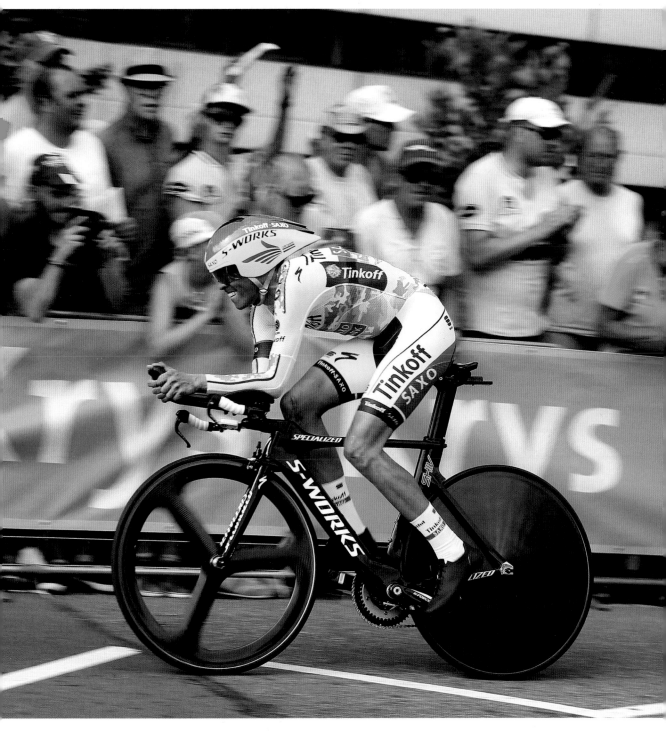

it like you would a golf ball. They create mini trips of airflow so it hangs onto the surface longer and, in turn, lowers drag.'

'Skinsuits are just really interesting,' Martin continues. 'Things like where the seams are placed and distribution of rough-to-smooth fabric can begin to be evaluated for a specific rider's anatomy and riding style, all with the aim of reducing the coefficient of drag.'

There's no Holy Grail when it comes to fabric manipulation. At the 2015 Tour de France, in the team time trial Movistar wore skinsuits with ribbed upper arms and shoulders. However, by the time stage one's team time trial came around at that year's Vuelta, Endura had replaced the stripe pattern with a new surface texture technology that used lots of small arrowhead-shaped protrusions to create frequent changes in texture. The aim of both designs was to delay separation of air from the suit to reduce drag and speed you up.

Reducing drag is also the aim of the NoPinz speedsuits and pockets. Instead of pinning race numbers to a suit, which creates a parachute effect, the British company created suits with a large transparent pocket integrated into the fabric at the rear for the race number to slip into. It's claimed that losing the billowing race number can save at least 3.5 watts, which if riding at 25mph for a 25-mile time trial could equate to a 20-second saving.

Lotto NL-Jumbo were sufficiently impressed to order a batch for the 2015 Tour de France, and reaped immediate dividends with two riders inside the top 10 at the 13.8km opening prologue – Jos van Emden fifth and Wilco Kelderman ninth: the lowest cumulative time for three riders of 46.06 minutes.

## Aerodynamic savings

UK cycle coach Joe Beer reveals the importance of gear selection on racing fast in the table below. Time savings are over a 40km time-trial course with a rider based on wind-tunnel testing in Brackley and track time at the Newport velodrome.

| TRADITIONAL GEAR | ADVANCED GEAR | TIME SAVING |
|---|---|---|
| Round fork | Aerodynamic fork | 30 seconds |
| Economy skinsuit | Custom-made | 30–60 seconds |
| Spoked wheels | Disc wheel plus tri-spoke | 60–90 seconds |
| Vented helmet | Aerodynamic helmet | 60–120 seconds |
| Handlebars | Aerobars | 45–60 seconds |
| No overshoes | Overshoes | 30 seconds |

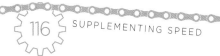

# ROAD-STAGE REFINEMENT

That attention to clothing detail has historically focused on time trials, but aero-dynamics aren't just for time trials. Every major clothing bike apparel brand now focuses on reducing drag over long road stages. The days of flapping cycle tops are long gone.

'In 2010 I remember asking Team Sky about the potential of wearing a skinsuit on the road,' says Greg Henderson, who now rides for Lotto-Soudal. 'Then Sky came straight back to me with these skinsuits with two pockets in the back. I think I rode the whole Giro in one. That's when aerodynamic road gear really started to take off.'

While Henderson's full-body skinsuit is rare for six hours in the saddle – it could become too hot and uncomfortable – more common is the jersey/short combo. Italian clothing brand Castelli, who clothe Cannondale-Garmin and riders of the calibre of Andrew Talansky, brought out their original Aero race jersey back in 2007. With advances in material technology, the body-hugging top purported to provide comfort but was tight enough to run slipshod through the air.

'Take the third incarnation of the Aero Race jersey, which we brought out when the Cervélo Test Team were launched in 2009,' says Richard Mardle, who works for Castelli in the UK. 'That was fast but since then the garment's evolved. The front panel, for instance, had a high level of Lycra to polyester for a slippery finish, but now has an equal balance for improved breathability and still allows the same performance gains due to fabric construction techniques. With the Aero Race 5.0 jersey, we saved 12 watts at 40km/h.'

Mardle highlights the dual aims of performance and comfort, which is clearly of benefit over 21 stages of racing. It's a point picked up on by Giant-Alpecin's Koen de Kort. 'It's now a combination of aerodynamics and comfort, and being warm or cool enough depending on the conditions,' he says. 'There's certainly a greater focus on aerodynamics these days – you won't find many riding around with zippers open anymore.'

When you're riding at an intense pace, the aerobic nature of the sport means you're producing a huge amount of perspiration. That's where wicking comes in (which we elaborate on in Chapter 11). Wicking refers to the process where a material takes sweat away from the body. Sports clothing manufacturers have been making this a priority for many years. Fit is key for good wicking.

'If a garment claims to be taking sweat away from the body (wicking), it needs to be in contact with the body,' says Dr Simon Hodder, an expert in thermal management in apparel at Loughborough University, England. 'But fit is vital. If a top's too baggy, it just won't wick properly, if at all. If it's too tight, that's not so much of an issue, though it can cause discomfort and lose its insulation properties.'

Which isn't a problem when it's hot. But thermal issues strike riders when riders reach the summit of a significant climb. The ambient temperature drops and a degree of insulation is what they're after. So a perfect-fitting top is what the riders need – one that can cool in the heat and keep them warm in the chilly winds. 'That's also where they might slip on a winter gilet or something similar,' says Simon Huntsman, head of R&D at Rapha, suppliers of kit to Team Sky. (That 'something similar' can include the age-old technique of stuffing newspapers beneath the riders' jerseys to reduce wind-chill. At neutral zones, individuals wandering around offloading newspapers to the *directeurs sportifs*' cars remains a common sight.)

There are further considerations when it comes to designing clothing for the Tour. Every rider will have some form of race nutrition buried in their rear pocket, be it gels, bars or real food. For domestiques, this can include numerous bottles for teammates. 'That's where the physical requirements of the garment comes in,' says Huntsman. 'For example, on a knit-based fabric, you need a certain amount of integrity in the fabric. For instance, when your pockets are loaded, you don't want it to sag. Along the sides, you want a bit more stretch and comfort so that you can reach the bars.'

And despite the aerodynamic evolution, that comfort remains key. In his autobiography *My Time*, Bradley Wiggins bemoans picking up the yellow jersey at the 2012 Critérium du Dauphiné ahead of the long time trial because of the uncomfortable leader's kit, which is always supplied by Le Coq Sportif at ASO races. 'Their skinsuits don't suit me because they have panels on the arms where the logo of Le Crédit Lyonnais, the race sponsor, is printed. The logo has to be printed a certain way so they put in the panel, which is stitched across the top of the biceps… It's uncomfortable because when I get into my tuck position, the stitching pulls my arms and I get a lot of cuts right into the flesh. It's purely down to my body shape.'

## SAFETY, COOLING AND SPEED

Not that long ago, little attention was paid to helmet aerodynamics when riding in a group – partly because helmets were only made mandatory in 2003 after the death of Andrei Kivilev – although it's speculated that riders often covered their vents with cling film for marginal benefits in a sprint or breakaway. What's certain is that less rudimentary vent covers have been used. The UCI banned detachable helmet covers in 2012, but not before Mark Cavendish had stormed to victory in the 2011 World Championships, his Specialized Prevail featuring a clear plastic cover. But that was a mere speedbump along the road to more aerodynamic road helmets.

Cavendish's plastic covering fast-tracked the industry to launch aerodynamic road helmets. This went against history because, typically, long road stages through a province like Brittany would see riders choose a vented helmet; if it was every man for himself against the clock in a time trial, a teardrop-shaped aero helmet that flowed into their backs would be worn. Then things changed in 2012 when Italian helmet manufacturers Kask, who supply Team Sky with their helmets, brought out the Bambino and Giro the Air Attack, regarded as the world's first aerodynamic road helmets.

Rob Wesson is director of helmet production creation at Giro and explains the concept behind aerodynamic road helmets. 'Whenever you ride, you have the wind coming at you, often with a 10° yaw angle. So the front of the helmet is very similar to a traditional time-trial helmet, from a thickness standpoint and the angle that it sweeps over the head.

'We kept the vents to a minimum because they disrupt airflow, and played around with where we could place the vents and still elicit breathability but not to the detriment of aerodynamics,' continues Wesson. 'We knew it had to be smaller, shorter, more compact on the head than a TT version, which can be cumbersome. So when we started doing our tests we had full TT helmets in our line-up to compare aero against road. So we have two extremes – TT helmet against road.

'TT helmets are faster, yes, but something like the Air Attack fits right in the middle. We get this impressive improvement in aerodynamics over normal vented helmets from factors like the sculpted and sharp edges.'

Sceptics would suggest that aerodynamic road helmets are merely another product of the bike industry to flog to consumers. Wesson argues otherwise. 'We have independent testing from BMC Racing whose results showed an improvement of 56 seconds. The teams are much smarter about their training these days. They know how to correlate power to speed to aerodynamics. They'll keep blogs and give great real-world feedback. We're not just a marketing machine trying to trick people.'

> ❛Whenever you ride, you have the wind coming at you, often with a 10° yaw angle. ❜
>
> **Rob WESSON,** *Giro*

Still, as Wesson says, the new wave of aerodynamic road helmets, like the Giant Rivet and Bontrager Ballista, aren't as fast as the traditional teardrop-shaped option used by Tour riders in a time trial – which are a proven piece of streamlined speed.

A benchmark study by Stephanie Sidelko of MIT in America compared 10 different aerodynamic time-trial helmets to a standard vented helmet. The helmets were used on a mannequin named Uri in a wind tunnel and the helmet was placed in three different positions – very close to the back with the rear of the helmet almost touching Uri's back; slightly away from Uri's back; and placed with Uri's head looking down and the tip straight up.

Sidelko showed that even the worst-performing aerodynamic helmet created less drag than its vented sibling, which is more breathable and lighter but creates more turbulent air because of those vents. Over a time trial and generating an average power output of 450 watts, the professional rider could conserve between 22.8 and 35.2 watts when selecting the non-vented teardrop at 0° yaw angle (in other words, wind hitting the rider face on). The more real-life 10° yaw (wind hitting the rider at 10° from face on) still witnessed power savings of between 21.3 and 29.1 watts.

The contribution of the helmet to a rider's total aerodynamic drag sits between 2 per cent and 8 per cent depending on its profile – things like positioning of vents and front profile of helmet – with further studies showing a TT version can realise savings of 90 seconds during a 40km time trial, an improvement of 3 per cent.

How aerodynamic helmets work is similar to aerodynamic road frames, encouraging laminar flow, though like the latest skinsuits, some also feature patches of rough to create minuscule surface turbulence so that the separation of the boundary layer from the surface is delayed. Some, like the Louis Garneau Vorttice helmet, have a dimpled finish like a golf ball for purportedly less drag.

'It's true that the full-on non-vented aerodynamic helmets are faster but that comes at a thermal cost,' says Wesson. Numerous studies into thermal effects of aerodynamic versus vented show that teardrop-shaped helmets lead to increased core and skin temperature, which results in greater metabolic cost. In other words, the rider gets too hot. That and the fact their pointy tails are hardly practical when riding in the peloton is why they're the preserve of shorter time trials only. As

▽ Movistar's Alejandro Valverde (L) and Nairo Quintana, both wearing Catlike's highly-vented helmets

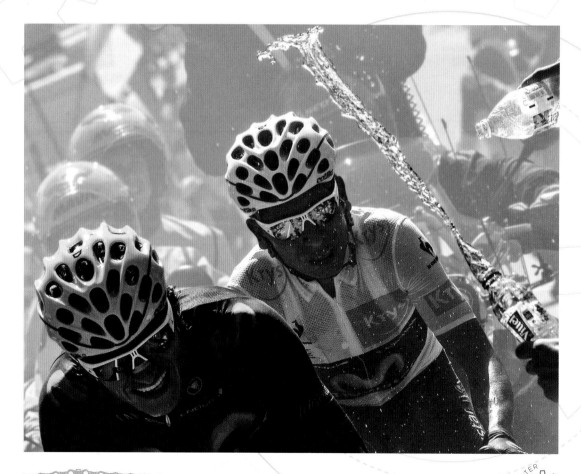

Wesson says, aerodynamic road helmets sit right in the middle: lacking the tail but with fewer vents than the traditional peloton chapeau.

And they also strike a balance in terms of heat transfer. A School of Aerospace study at RMTI University showed that the pitch of vents has a notable effect on heat transfer, indicating that when the vents were pitched at 45°, all helmets showed lower head temperature than at 90°. Positioning of the vents (front and back) on the helmet is also important as incoming air enters into the head surface to remove the heat through the back.

'Heat management is more common with vented helmets but when working with McLaren on our latest aerodynamic road helmet that optimises the shape so that the rider can bury their head or tuck in, we included side vents like they'd use in Formula One,' says Chris Yu, aerodynamics engineer with Specialized. 'This increases ventilation, though a bonus is that we discovered it reduces drag.'

# GRAPHENE – THE MAGIC MATERIAL

But it's not just aerodynamic-led designs that are reshaping headwear. Use of technically–advanced materials are becoming commonplace. Spanish bike helmet manufacturer Catlike protects the heads of the likes of Nairo Quintana and Alejandro Valverde at Movistar. While the outer shell of their top-end Mixino helmet uses traditional polycarbonate sheets, the inner cage is graphene.

'The head's protected by an aramid cage [man-made fibres that are charac-terised by relatively rigid polymer chains, which create a strong structure] with poly-styrene balls stuck to it and heat-treated and pressurised,' says Ana Villa, Catlike's European sales manager. 'We also add graphene.' This is quite a coup for Catlike as they're the first helmet manufacturer to market with this wonder material, one that conducts electricity better than copper (admittedly not useful on a helmet), is more pliable than rubber and 200 times stronger than steel but six times lighter.

'Graphene is a single sheet of carbon atoms,' says Dr Aravind Vijayaraghavan, lecturer in nanomaterials at Manchester University. 'Each carbon atom is connected to three other carbon atoms via very strong covalent bonds. This structure makes graphene extremely strong and stretchable.'

Graphene was discovered in 2004 when Manchester University's Andre Geim engaged in an experiment that involved peeling away layers from a graphite pencil with sticky tape. The monotonous stripping paid off, as the team eventually isolated a one-atom-thick substance that was strong, light, and an excellent conductor of heat and electricity. This groundbreaking discovery led to Geim receiving the 2010 Nobel Prize for Physics. But despite the plaudits, its evolution to the mass market has been hampered by an inability to produce it cost effectively and on a commer-cial scale. Until now.

'We source graphene from one of the only companies in the world who can produce it in industrial quantities. They're called Graphenea,' says Villa. 'It makes the helmet very strong and very light. We use it in the soles of some of our bicycle shoes, too.'

When the process of mass graphene production becomes even more refined, it's clear that a world of cycling possibilities awaits. Its lightness and strength are perfect for frame material; conductivity could see electronic groupset batteries integrated into the frame; its pliability and transparency could forge foldable touch screens that wrap around a rider's bars.

Catlike are also innovators when it comes to bespoke helmets for the leading Movistar riders, like Quintana and Valverde, using a cranial scanner to map the rider's skull dimensions before manufacturing their custom model.

'The link-up with Movistar has not only been a commercial success but has driven innovation,' adds Villa. 'We've worked with the riders and the sports scientists at Granada University, testing and refining helmets in the wind tunnel and on CFD.'

Like bikes, the wind tunnel and computational fluid dynamics (CFD) software is helping helmet manufacturers shave the odd watt here and there in pursuit of speed. That was Chris Boardman's aim when he was part of British Cycling's noted Secret Squirrel club, which was assembled by Team Sky boss Dave Brailsford (see the 'Secret Squirrel' box on page 110). Boardman was part of the team that delivered British Cycling 28 advances in aspects like performance analysis and clothing between January 2010 and the successful London Olympics.

> ❝Electronic groupsets have made a big difference in time trials.❞
>
> Alex DOWSETT, *Movistar*

Integral to advancing industry knowledge was bringing in experts from a non-cycling background, with Boardman citing Rob Lewis of TotalSim in England as one of the key recruits. TotalSim are global leaders in CFD application, beginning with the F1 industry at British American Racing and then Honda, before applying it to other aerodynamic-seeking sectors that included British Cycling.

Lewis helped drive the sport forward but not everything passed UCI rules. 'I remember one of the first things Rob created was what we called "the dangler",' says Boardman. 'He had somebody's aero helmet with a piece of string and ball attached, both hanging in front of the rider. He asked, "Can I do that?" I said "No, but why would you want to anyway?" He explained that though there might be a localised loss due to the disrupted airflow, it might lead to net gains once the air reached the helmet. Stuff like that helped determine optimum placements of bike computers.'

Boardman adds that British Cycling also toyed with ideas like sewing sequins into skinsuits, the aim being greater aerodynamics by disrupting airflow. But Chris Hoy dressed like Liberace sadly never took off.

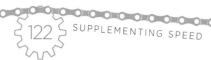

# THE CHARGED PELOTON

Neither did Mavic's electronic groupset back in 1992 (the groupset is the moving parts of the bike: chainring, cranks, chain, derailleurs and brakes). A full 16 years before Shimano launched the Di2, Mavic created the world's first electronic groupset. Chris Boardman used it and was a fan. 'The beauty of the ZAP groupset was that the battery only had to send a signal to the rear mechanism where a solenoid [a coil wound into a tightly packed helix] engaged the jockey wheel and the rider's pedalling action changed the gear. It meant the battery could be tiny,' he told *US Peloton* magazine.

The advantages of mechanical-free, electronic gear shift systems like Shimano's Di2 and Campagnolo's EPS include: more precise, quicker gear changes; reduced chain wear; and the facility to allow multiple locations for shifters, making the process of swapping cogs as simple as the press of a button.

That's the ideal. Unfortunately, with the ZAP you could only shift one sprocket at a time – not nearly enough for the sprinters – though that was the least of the problems. Reliability issues, including waterproofing failure, killed retailer and consumer confidence and, despite ONCE and RMO using it in the Tour, the ZAP was taken off the market in 1994.

Mavic tried again in 1999 with the wireless Mektronic, but again, issues like limited gear range meant it failed to gain a foothold in the wider cycling community and the product was soon dropped. 'Maybe we were too early to market,' says Mavic's global PR manager Michel Lethenet.

Mavic are to be applauded for their innovative efforts, especially as it took the industry until 2009 before electronic groupsets began appearing again in the professional ranks, seen first at that year's Tour of California via Columbia High Road, Garmin Slipstream and Rabobank. Despite their innovation, price and maintenance has held back their recruitment by recreational riders. It's a different story for the professionals in 2016.

'Electronic groupsets have made a big difference in time trials,' says Movistar's Alex Dowsett. 'It might not make a huge difference in England because most of the time trials are up and down a dual carriageway. You come out of a country lane on the aerobars, onto the dual carriageway and away you go.

'But on the WorldTour, time trials can be highly technical. That's where they really pay off. To be able to shift mid-corner and not have to think about the gear you'll need to be in on exit saves time. Also, when coming off the start line, if you don't have electric gears, you have to think about do I start in a big gear, accelerate out of the saddle or do you start in a smaller gear and stay on the saddle. Either way, a mechanical can cost you two seconds straight away off the start ramp. Electronic is a no-brainer.'

Whereas mechanical shifters required some dexterous – and at times forceful – fingers and thumbs, electronic groupsets use a button. As Dowsett said, that means the professional rider can stay in an aerodynamic tuck longer. In the world of marginal gains, that could make the difference.

Time trials are where electronic gears come into their own – unlike long, flat stages, where there's no advantage over mechanical because, like cruising on the motorway, gear changes are rare. 'It has a big impact on the classics, though, as it did on stage three of the 2015 Tour,' says Giant-Alpecin's Koen de Kort, referring to the 159.5km stage from Anvers to Huy that concluded on the Mur de Huy, which earlier in 2015 provided the finish line for Flèche Wallonne. 'The defining characteristics of the classics, especially the Ardennes, are short, steep climbs. With Di2 [Shimano's electronic groupset], you go up a steep climb in a low gear and then have to really accelerate over the top of the climb. You need to rapidly move from a low to high gear, and it's that bit quicker with Di2. That can make a difference as if you lose the pack and its drafting benefits and are left on your own, you'll drift back because you have no energy-saving pack protection.'

Electronic gears are a relatively new weapon in the professional rider's armoury but a saddle is as old as the bike itself. And at its heart, the saddle hasn't changed: its primary aim is still comfort – which is just as well for the Tour riders who spend 90 hours on it.

# PLATFORM FOR POWER AND SUCCESS

Italian brand fi'zi:k provide saddles for Movistar, Orica GreenEdge, FDJ, Team Sky and BMC Racing. They know their saddles. Fi'zi:k's racing manager Nicolo Ildos certainly does – and reveals there's a great deal of science and complexity beneath Froome and van Garderen's buttocks.

'We do pressure mapping to calculate where the rider's weight is distributed,' he says. 'We did a lot of testing at universities, too, and also made a special tool to simulate riding up and downhill. Both of these affect your sitting position.'

Fi'zi:k's range of high-performance saddles is vast. Chris Froome uses the Antares 00, which comes in at a lightweight 135g; Philippe Gilbert the Volta, featuring an inverted-U-shaped profile, which increases comfort for riders who move around a lot; and Thibaut Pinot the Arione, designed for flexible riders who enjoy an aggressive racing position.

'Many of the saddles also include carbon, which results in more efficient power transfer between the moving rider and pedals,' adds Ildos. 'It makes them very stiff, but stiffness isn't great for everyone. So we offer multiple options in our range because everyone rides differently.'

Stiffness isn't ideal over the cobbled classics or the cobbled stages of the Tour. That's why many riders, including Bradley Wiggins and Geraint Thomas, had

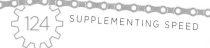

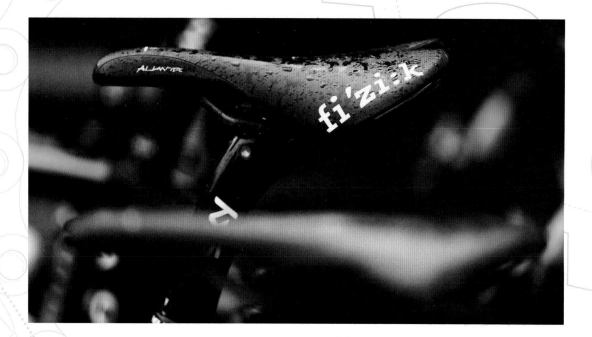

△ Fi'zi:k support
many WorldTour
teams including Sky

custom-made Arione saddles made, which featured extra padding for more comfort.

'That's rare, though,' says Ildos. 'Around 99 per cent of the time, professionals use off-the-shelf saddles. We have such a wide range that we can accommodate many riders. I do remember one special case, though, when we made a saddle especially for Ivan Basso. He had really bad inflammation from saddle sores and needed antibiotics. It was painful.'

But like all of the gear adopted by professional riders, each will have their own steer, their own idiosyncrasies, of how they apply that garment, helmet or saddle to their own performance. 'Take Tony Gallopin,' says teammate at Lotto-Soudal Greg Henderson. 'He's always changing his saddle height. Always. That's not unusual for a rider from the track but rare for a pure roadie.'

Tinkering isn't unusual; riders like Bernard Hinault were famed for their attention to detail. But riders today are refining their performance with the most scientifically proven equipment in the history of cycling. The advent of wind tunnels and software to gauge the drag on an object has created a multimillion industry of cycle clothing, helmets and componentry, all proclaiming to go faster or hit the scales lighter than ever before. While integration is the future of bike design, the same is true when it comes to an increasing focus on bespoke gear. As 3D printers become more affordable, constructing a garment that matches the specific dimensions of any rider on the team will become as standardised as having a bike fit or taking a fitness test. Whether that'll make riding at 2,000m any easier is debatable – and that's where we go next on our quest to uncover the science behind the Tour de France.

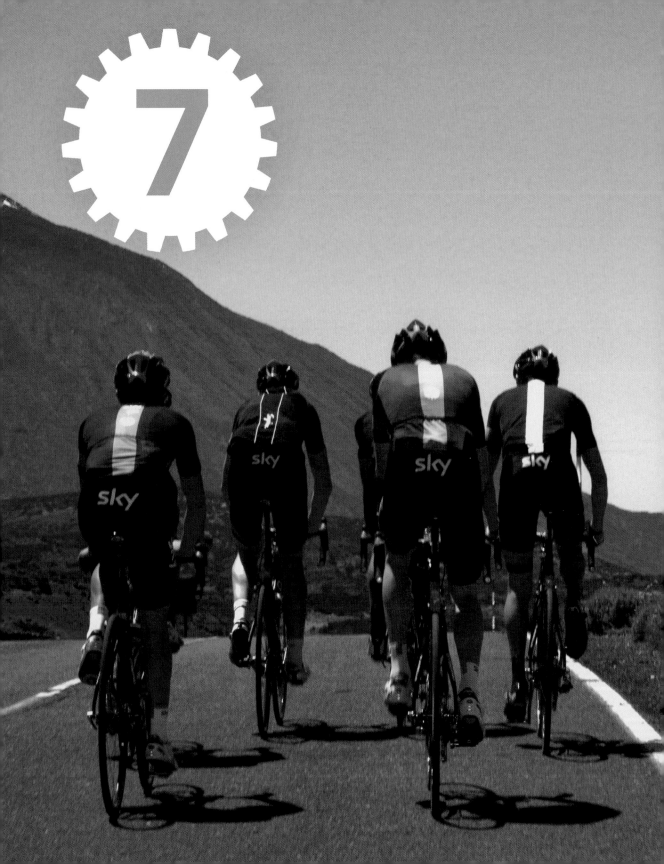

# IN SEARCH OF OXYGEN

The Parador Hotel at the summit of Mount Teide in Tenerife is cycling's equivalent of the celebrity-filled Chateau Marmont in Los Angeles. Over the years, professional teams including Team Sky, Tinkoff Sport and Astana have gravitated to the Parador – the only hotel in Tenerife's national park – in search of seclusion, sun and air – or lack of it. The peak of Mount Teide is 3,178m high, making it the highest mountain peaking out of Spanish territory, but it's the roads situated around 2,300m that are of more interest to the professional peloton. (As illustrated in the build-up to the 2014 Tour when Chris Froome took to Twitter to admonish cycling's governing body, the UCI: 'Three major contenders staying on Mt Teide and no out-of-competition tests for the past two weeks. Very disappointing.' He was referring to Vincenzo Nibali, who went on to dominate that year's Tour, Alberto Contador and himself.)

'The aim of altitude training at places like Tenerife is to lift elite riders' performance by around 2 per cent,' says Sam Rees, performance specialist at the Altitude Centre in London, whose clients include British Cycling and a number of professional riders. In cycling's world of marginal gains, 2 per cent is huge, and would have seen 2014 33rd-place finisher Tom Dumoulin jump to becoming the holder of the yellow jersey.

Clearly performance is more complex than just sitting at the top of a mountain during your training. But the very effective premise behind altitude training is relatively simple: by exposing a cyclist to an environment that's low in oxygen, the body will adapt by becoming more efficient at transporting and using oxygen. And as cycling is predominantly an aerobic sport, oxygen rules.

At sea level, air contains 21 per cent oxygen. It's the same at 2,000m, 3,000m and so on. The difference is, as you go higher, the air becomes less compressed, thinner and harder to breathe. So while Froome and Kennaugh can swim in the Atlantic Ocean off Tenerife (i.e. at sea level or 0m) inhaling 21 per cent oxygen, when they cycle to around 2,300m above sea level, the *effective* oxygen percentage

◁ Team Sky on one of their frequent altitude training camps in Tenerife

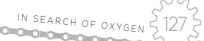

decreases to below 16 per cent.

While it might feel like torture for the cyclists the benefits have been shown to be enormous. 'Studies have shown that training at altitude: increases $VO_2$ max by anything from 3 to 8 per cent; decreases heart rate, both at rest and during exercise; increases myoglobin, the muscle protein; reduces lactic acid build-up; and facilitates greater production of EPO from the kidneys,' says Rees.

Ahh, EPO – the elephant in the room of any professional cyclist. EPO, or erythropoietin, is the hormone that in its synthetic form became as at home in Lance Armstrong's fridge as a pint of milk. The natural form of EPO is produced in the kidneys and stimulates the production of red blood cells, which picks up oxygen from the lungs and transports it to the working muscles. The simple equation is: the more red blood cells, the greater oxygen, the harder and longer you can work.

'With altitude training, essentially we're looking for the same results as the blood dopers were; in other words, boosting aspects like haematocrit,' says Dr Jonathan Baker, sports scientist at Team Dimension Data. 'The difference is, it's legal.'

Haematocrit is the percentage of red blood cells in your blood – the remainder is blood plasma, which is 95 per cent water. In 1997, the UCI implemented blood testing to deter the alleged use of rhEPO (synthetic EPO) by setting the upper limit as 50 per cent. In accordance with their desire to limit potential image-damaging results, the UCI President Hein Verbruggen stressed the test acted as a health check and a positive test didn't imply rhEPO use. 'Riders would be suspended until their levels returned to an acceptable level,' a UCI statement read.

Marco Pantani's career was peppered with such 'high moments'. In 1999 Pantani was leading the Giro d'Italia with just one mountain stage remaining when a blood test at Madonna di Campiglio showed a reading of 52 per cent. Disqualification followed, as did a two-week break for levels to dip under 50 per cent.

Haematocrit levels are no longer the primary focus of anti-doping. That's now left to the biological blood passport, which looks at blood profiles over time rather than isolated incidents. (See the 'Blood Passport' box on page 140 for more information.) However, Boulder-based altitude training outfit Higher Peak have suggested a rise of around 10 per cent is possible with effective altitude training. This would see someone with a haematocrit level of 45 per cent rise to around 50 per cent, theoretically meaning they could deliver 10 per cent more oxygen with every heartbeat.

While the spectre of illegally raising haematocrit levels remains through EPO micro-dosing, as cited in the UCI's 2015 CIRC report, unless a professional rider is blessed like Eero Mäntyranta, altitude work is the widely accepted norm used by professional teams to increase haematocrit numbers.

Finnish skier Mäntyranta won two cross-country skiing gold medals at the

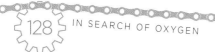

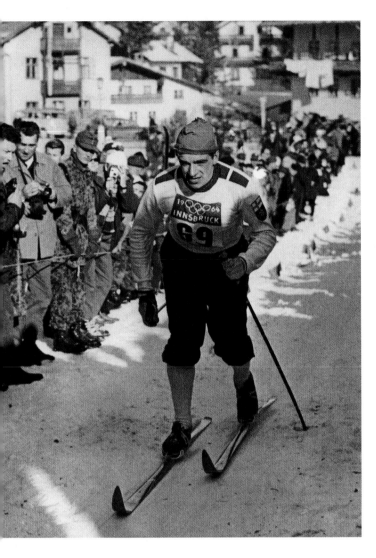

1964 Winter Olympics. Mäntyranta followed a similar diet to his contemporaries, trained the same way and wasn't exposed to the marginal gains that populate elite-level sport in 2015. But he had one clear advantage over his rivals: his oxygen-carrying haemoglobin levels naturally measured 236g per litre of blood at their peak compared to a usual range of 140–180g per litre. This blessed him with a haematocrit level of over 60 per cent.

Researchers at the University of Helsinki, Finland, in 1993 focused on the Mäntyranta family and observed that 29 members, including Eero, all had a genetic mutation that affected the EPO receptor, meaning their bone marrow produced red blood cells without being stimulated by the hormone EPO. In short, he was genetically predisposed to endurance sport.

Riders like Marco Pantani cast a suspicious shadow over any rider who is genetically blessed with having a haematocrit level over the UCI limit. One such rider was Britain's Charly Wegelius, *directeur sportif* at Cannondale-Garmin.

△ Gold-medal-winning cross-country skiing Eero Mantyranta naturally had huge levels of haemoglobin

'When I was coaching Charly as a youngster, we had regular blood tests in case the riders fell ill and the doctors needed a baseline to test against,' says coach Ken Matheson. 'During that time we began to realise something was going on in the peloton [with EPO]. The 50 per cent rule came in so I had a look at my riders. It was 46, 43 … Charly came in at 52. He was only 16 at the time.'

Wegelius progressed through the ranks and was selected to race for Great Britain. Matheson recalls contacting then team manager John Herety to inform him – that, if he was tested, he could well be over that threshold. Not long after, Wegelius was pulled from the 2003 Tour of Lombardy. 'I thought, "Shit – why wasn't anything done?" I phoned Charly and he said it hadn't been sorted.'

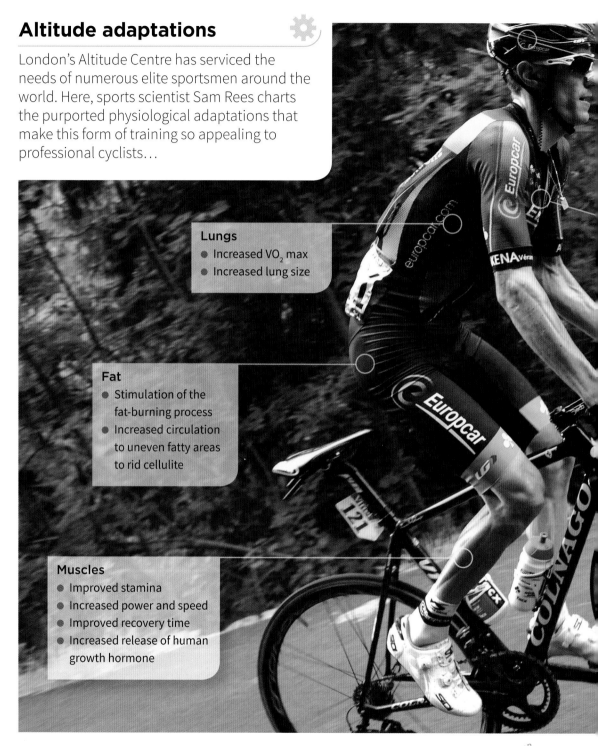

# Altitude adaptations

London's Altitude Centre has serviced the needs of numerous elite sportsmen around the world. Here, sports scientist Sam Rees charts the purported physiological adaptations that make this form of training so appealing to professional cyclists…

**Lungs**
- Increased $VO_2$ max
- Increased lung size

**Fat**
- Stimulation of the fat-burning process
- Increased circulation to uneven fatty areas to rid cellulite

**Muscles**
- Improved stamina
- Increased power and speed
- Improved recovery time
- Increased release of human growth hormone

### Brain

- Up-regulated glucose transport activity with an increase of GLUT1 – the food the brain requires
- Protected from oxidative stress
- Increased potency of adaptive sleep
- Improved concentration span

### Heart

- Decreased heart rate both at rest and during exercise
- Decreased blood pressure, both at rest and during exercise
- Greater stroke volume – amount of blood pumped from heart during each contraction

### Blood

- Increases in capillary density and improved circulation
- Elevated nitric oxide levels to release more oxygen to the working muscles
- Elevated vascular endothelial growth factor (VEGF) – the cells that make up the inside of blood vessel)
- Natural erythropoietin (EPO) production – a hormone manufactured by the kidney that stimulates red blood cell production
- Increased reticulocyte production – young red blood cells that are formed in the bone marrow
- Increased haemoglobin levels – the part of the red blood cell that carries oxygen
- Increased number and efficiency of mitochondria – the body's principal energy producer
- Reduced blood lactate at a given workload
- Improved blood buffering capability, meaning exercise-derived acidic levels remain low enough not to impair muscle contraction

### Cells

- Increased myoglobin (the muscle protein) levels
- Increase in enzymes involved in the metabolism of fat
- Reduction in lactate acid build-up
- Increase in oxidative enzymes in the mitochondria
- Increase in ATP activity (adenosine triphosphate) – the cell's energy source

◁ France's Pierre Rolland rides in a breakaway during the 138km nineteenth stage of the 2015 Tour de France, between Saint-Jean-de-Maurienne and La Toussuire

Thankfully, Matheson had 'illegally' retained all of his blood tests (you weren't supposed to retain them), providing the evidence needed to clear Wegelius of any wrongdoing. In the process of defending his athlete, Matheson and his team also tested Charly's father in the hope of adding further weight to their genetic defence. He came in at 56.

# HEIGHT LIMIT

Italian Marco Pinotti is coach at BMC Racing. He retired from racing the professional circuit at the end of 2013 but not before he'd had spells in the *maglia rosa* at the 2007 and 2011 Giro d'Italia, as well as winning six Italian national time-trial titles. Pinotti proved a popular racer, not just because of his competitive exploits but because he was a vocal opponent of doping. The engineering graduate was known as Italy's voice of reason through the height of the *omerta*, and acquired the nickname the Cycling Professor from his progressive search for legal improvements. On his quest for more speed, Pinotti's consumed many a mile at thin air.

'It's hard work,' he says. 'Your breathing's restricted; in fact, it feels like you're breathing through a straw. But that's an unavoidable truth. Science has shown that you need to head over 1,500m to "enjoy" the benefits of altitude training, though the closer you get to around 2,000–2,300m, the better.'

You might ask why not 3,000m? Or 5,000m? Surely the adaptations that are so beneficial to a cyclist's performance will be greater the thinner the air? Ask Peter Sagan why. The green jersey winner at the 2012–2014 Tours is one of the more colourful characters in the peloton, and moved from Cannondale to Tinkoff Sport at the end of 2014 for a reported annual salary of €4 million. The ink had barely dried on his three-year contract before Sagan had experienced team-bonding Tinkoff style – an ascent of Mount Kilimanjaro. 'I was okay up until the 5,000m mark,' says Sagan. 'That's when I began to have problems with headaches and balance. At the top I vomited. It was like having a hangover.'

We're sure the charismatic Sagan's never touched alcohol … but this drowsy and lethargic feeling is a situation that's compounded (ironically) by his and his contemporaries' fitness levels. 'Professional cyclists would have trained their body to extract all the oxygen available to them, whatever level they're training or racing,' explains Rees. 'What happens at high altitude is that your muscles take every oxygen atom they can, meaning there's little left in the bloodstream – certainly less than with the recreational riders we see. So while that's good for working muscles, it can leave you nauseous and light-headed.'

That's why that figure of around 2,000–2,300m is seemingly the Holy Grail of altitude training: not high enough to leave you vomiting, not so low that you don't adapt. Tenerife hits that perfectly. 'Our team went there in February,' says Pinotti. 'It's the only place you can logistically go at that time of year because of the

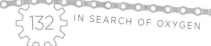

weather. Throughout the year, many of the team also visit Lake Tahoe in California (1,900m) and Livigno in Italy (1,816m), while Tejay [van Garderen] lives in Boulder, Colorado (around 1,700m). We probably do two or three altitude camps a year.'

Despite the prospect of creating a team of divorcees, it begs the question: if altitude stimulates such beneficial physiological changes, why not commit Froome, Nibali and the rest to all-year-round altitude camps, only releasing them from the Parador to satisfy their competitive urges?

'That's down to intensity of training,' says Baker. 'Because there's less oxygen the further you climb, your power output is lower. Let's say a rider like Tyler Farrar is generating 300 watts at sea level, the power output to achieve the same speed at altitude might be 350 watts. So while their blood levels improve, with regard to reticulocyte production (young red blood cells) and haemoglobin levels (the part of the red blood cell that carries oxygen), their muscles actually weaken. It's why altitude training is such a tricky balance to get right.'

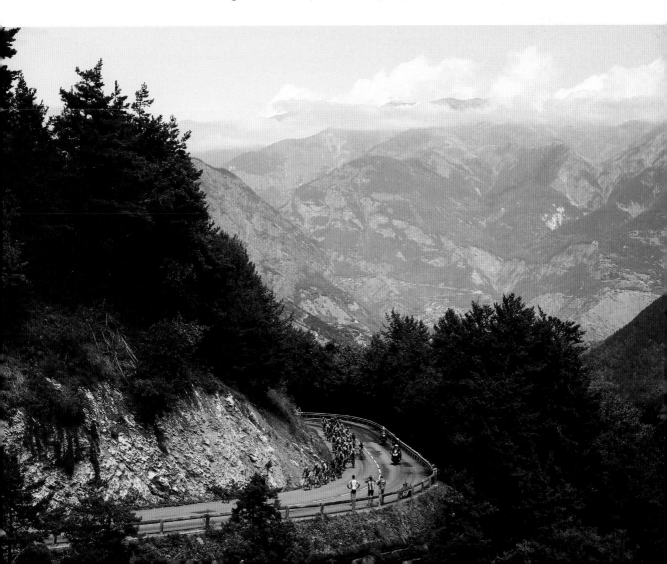

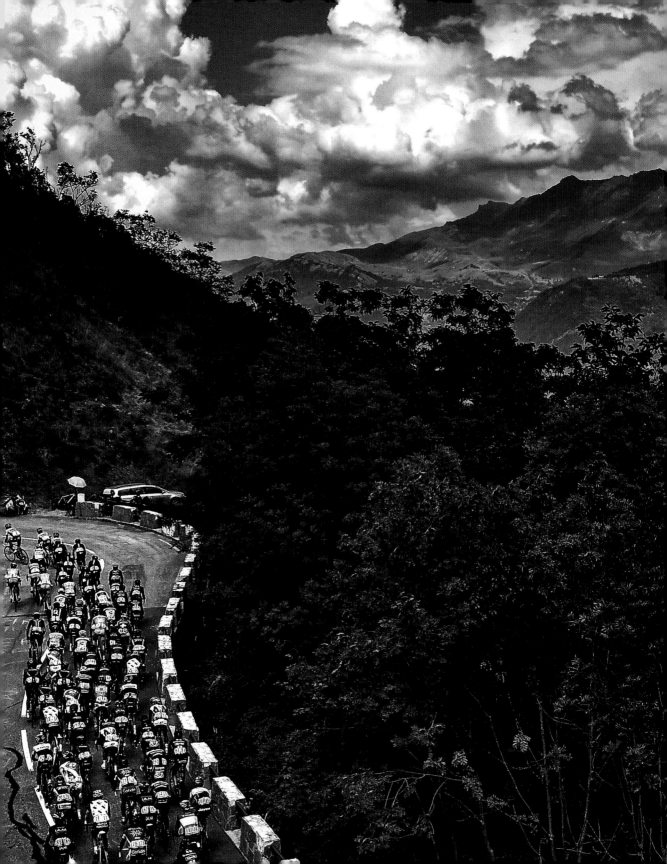

⊲ The pack rides during the 138km nineteenth stage of the 2015 Tour de France, between Saint-Jean-de-Maurienne and La Toussuire

That weakening of muscles is down to low-oxygen conditions at altitude triggering your adrenal glands to increase cortisol production. Cortisol is a catabolic hormone, meaning it breaks down muscle for energy in a process called catabolism. High cortisol levels cause your body to go from a muscle-building state to one of muscle breakdown. Cardiac output (amount of blood pumped by the heart each minute) and blood flow to the muscles also decreases, leading to a loss in muscular power.

Still, the pros seemingly outweigh the cons and altitude training is prevalent across every Tour team. Where the teams are less unified is the most effective application method. There are two contrasting theories: live high/train high or live high/train low. Let's delve a little deeper.

The focus on altitude training became popular during and after the 1968 Olympics in Mexico. Mexico City, which hosted track and field events, stands at just over 2,200m. Many federations spent time and resources studying the effects of altitude on elite athletes in the run-up to the Games, and a new sector of performance analysis was born.

Living and training at altitude was first tried because it made sense practically. Riders would experience full altitude exposure as they lived, ate, trained and slept high. Like subsequent research into altitude training, the advantages remain equivocal. A 1975 study had male-distance runners spend three weeks training at 2,300m before testing their baseline values back down at sea level. The results showed no increase in aerobic capacity. A further study by Daniels and Olridge in 1970 realised up to a 5 per cent increase in $VO_2$ max values with an average 3 per cent boost in the runners' three-mile times. On the downside, as Team Dimension Data's John Baker alluded to, training intensity was hampered.

In the late 1990s, athletes began to play around with the idea of sleeping at altitude but training at sea level, the idea being they'd physiologically adapt while they slept but could still train to a high intensity by day.

A study by the AIS (Australian Institute of Sport – a hotbed of sport science) compared a control group of seven athletes who lived and trained at sea level against a group who trained at sea level but slept for 23 nights in simulated altitude of 3,000m (see page 145 on altitude tents). The scientists took muscle biopsies from each athlete after the 24-day training period – unusual in itself as, not surprisingly, athletes aren't overly keen on losing cells from muscles – and discovered that $VO_2$ peak in the non-control group fell for the same amount of work (meaning they were more economical) while muscle-buffering capacity increased by 18 per cent (meaning they could sprint harder and longer). In essence, they found work easier than the control group.

'For many, living high and training low is the gold standard,' says the Altitude Centre's Sam Rees. 'You find that many riders will use this method because it's the most efficient way of incorporating altitude training without affecting the intensity

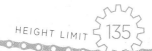

too much.' Though Rees espouses the benefits of an altitude tent (more later), they can't simulate the physical sensation of climbing a mountain. That's why professional teams continue to attend training camps up high, though are creative with their training plans.

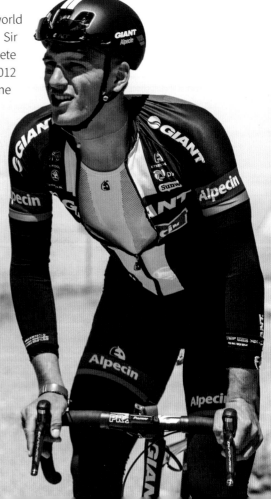

## ALTITUDE PROTOCOLS

Prior to the 2015 Tour de France, Giant-Alpecin held a three-week altitude camp in the Sierra Nevada, near Granada, Spain. The mountain range's highest peak is the Mulhacen, at 3,480m, though Marcel Kittel and John Degenkolb's team didn't train over 2,000m.

Attending the camp was Koen de Kort, who made his fifth appearance at the Tour in 2015. De Kort is part of Kittel's lead-out train and was happy to deconstruct the altitude camp. 'We sleep at altitude but often we'll head down to nearer sea level,' he says, in a Dutch accent tinged with Antipodean flavour ('the result of an Australian fiancée'). 'We'll train down there for the day and then be driven back up to our accommodation. That's the norm, though that will be broken up with altitude training two or three days a week.'

It's a template followed by professional teams the world over, including Team Sky. In his autobiography *My Time*, Sir Bradley Wiggins recalls the lengths he and head of athlete performance Tim Kerrison went to in pursuit of the 2012 *maillot jaune*. 'We'd done 4,000m of climbing and had one more 25-minute effort to go … We were at 1,500m altitude and were going to 2,200m. We'd ride one minute at 550 watts, basically prologue power, which you can sustain for a few minutes, then four minutes at threshold torque – 50rpm at threshold, maybe 400–440 watts depending on altitude, which is bloody hard to do because riding in the big ring, say 53 × 16 gear, at threshold on a climb, is like going up a steep hill in your car with your foot to the floor in fourth.' Wiggins and crew did it five times and it clearly worked.

It's relevant to note that Wiggins's most intense session came at the end of the altitude camp. According to Pinotti, that matches the science. 'One of the primary physiological adaptations to improve performance is down to increasing blood volume,' he says. 'But it takes minimum 10 days – if not 12–13 – for the body to adapt. That's when you might be able to train more intensively. Still, you wouldn't be able to match the intensity of sea level. You would, however, probably ride for longer, though that's more to do with the rider having no distractions like family or life-load.'

A simple method the elites employ to monitor these adaptations is via a heart rate monitor. When the riders first head to altitude, the immediate struggle for air means heart rate rises by between five and ten beats per minute. Over seven to ten days, as the body adapts, this elevated heart rate returns to normal.

'This is highly individual, though,' adds Pinotti. 'The more often you altitude train, the less time it takes to adapt. Your body has a kind of altitude memory.'

Pinotti suggests that altitude training every two months is optimum. Of course, the WorldTour calendar, which begins with the Tour Down Under in January and concludes with Lombardy in October, means this often isn't practical, and is why altitude training is often immediately followed with a race.

'We often go to altitude camp in preparation for the spring classics, which means heading high right before Tirreno-Adriatico,' says Pinotti. 'The knock-on effect is that the riders who were at altitude may start Tirreno in poor condition but will improve over the week and be strong come the classics. By then they'll be receiving the benefits of altitude training and not the lethargic side effects.'

It's a sentiment echoed by Kort. 'After the Sierra Nevada camp finishes, we head straight to the Tour of Switzerland. Now, this'll mean the start of the race will be a nightmare but it's worth it as the effects from altitude will carry over to the Tour de France.'

Professional cyclists race for around 80 days a year. That's mere child's play compared to the likes of Eddy Merckx who'd regularly rack up 120 days' worth of competition per annum but it's still enough to make altitude training and racing a tricky balancing act.

As Kort says, in the build-up to July's Tour de France, many riders will attend an altitude camp and then head for some last-minute race prep in Switzerland. The majority of contenders, however, head to the Critérium du Dauphiné. The race runs over eight days and features several mountainous stages. It finishes three weeks before the Tour, providing the perfect platform for some 'competitive sharpening'. It also leaves the riders time for altitude training before tapering for the early July start of the Tour.

'That three-week window is usually enough for the top riders to squeeze in another altitude camp and is often why the GC contenders will race the Dauphiné rather than in Switzerland, which finishes a week after the Dauphiné,' says Pinotti. 'If your form's growing, you can hit altitude and tick off a series of long climbs.

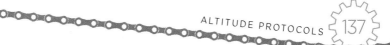

There'll also be time for one or two days of speedwork.'

'The problem is,' adds Brent Bookwalter, the BMC domestique who was part of the team that helped Cadel Evans to his 2011 Tour triumph, 'altitude training is so variable. One year I've seen a positive response from living high and training low. Twelve months later I'll follow the same protocol and the results haven't been anywhere near as good.'

That real-life inconsistency's reflected in the labs. In 2012, Indiana University exercise physiologist Robert Chapman subjected six elite distance runners to a 'live high, train low' altitude training programme in Arizona over the course of 28 days. The athletes lived at 2,150m and trained at 1,000m, following a series of sessions of varying intensities and duration.

The results showed that the athletes performed best within 48 hours of landing back down at sea level … or 18 to 22 days after. 'The problem is, there is little scientific evidence to show why these opinions are valid,' Chapman wrote, though he then suggested that the delayed improvement could have been down to a concept called ventilator acclimatisation. 'At altitude, a person breathes more, and that extra breathing stays with you when you come back down from altitude. Extra breathing uses more muscles, more energy and the body has to work more to regulate blood flow.' Over time, that settles down and you benefit from the adaptations.

If controlled studies can't agree on the perfect length of training camps and when you peak back down at sea level, it's no surprise that there's no set altitude menu. Professional cyclists are sensitive to change, especially if it's proved successful in the past. That's why altitude followed by the Dauphiné is a common combination.

What's more certain is that a species who live their lives in a perpetual state of hunger – so much so that former Classics specialist Sean Kelly entitled his autobiography *Hunger* (and not just about his competitive appetite) – will be even hungrier when training at altitude.

'At altitude, your body works harder just to perform simple functions like breathing,' says Pinotti. 'This raises your metabolism, so if you normally burn 3,000 calories a day, you might burn 3,300 calories at altitude. And in my personal experience, you're seeking these extra calories in the form of carbohydrates.'

Pinotti's craving of carbohydrates over fats as the major fuel source is supported by a band of … Andean mice. Research led by Marie-Pierre Schippers of McMaster University in Canada examined the metabolic processes of mountain-dwelling mice indigenous to the Andes, who resided at an altitude of around 4,000m above sea level. At that height, the breath inhaled by the Andean mice contained 40 per cent less oxygen than their sea-level cousins.

The researchers observed that the Andean mice metabolised significantly more energy from carbohydrates than fats. That's down to carbohydrates supplying 15 per cent more energy than fats for the same amount of oxygen.

While professional cyclists aren't scaling those heights, there'd still be a

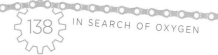

# Testing procedure

○ 'When you perform well, you're always tested,' says Giant-Shimano's manager Iwan Spekenbrink. Spekenbrink's right, with the stage and overall winner guaranteed a visit to doping control as well as their chasers. 'The goal of our athlete biological passport is to test riders a minimum of three times out-of-competition,' says Cycling Anti-Doping Foundation manager Olivier Banuls.

When you bear in mind that there were 17 WorldTour teams in 2015 with a maximum of 30 professional riders, that's 1,530 tests. As the UCI undertake over 4,000 out-of-competition tests, the UCI is hitting its target, though concedes that extra resource would make the system tighter.

When it comes to urine or blood collection, every sample is accompanied by an athlete questionnaire with Banuls stressing that athletes are asked to reveal if they've been at altitude within the past two weeks as this can affect the figures. This is corroborated by ADAMS (Anti-Doping Administration and Management System), which requires athletes to specify where there'll be for an hour a day, seven days a week, for up to three months, for random drug testing.

Though blood tests are a more reliable and detailed method of searching for illegal performance enhancers, urine tests are the practical norm during an event. Which is why John Degenkolb and co. have undergone this urinary test procedure many times over:

● The doping control officer or chaperone informs the rider they're to accompany them to the doping control building. Only under the following circumstances can the rider delay proceedings: victory ceremony; media commitments; further competitions; warm-down; medical treatment; locating a representative/interpreter; obtaining photo ID. The athlete is kept under strict observation at all times.

● A urine sample is provided in view of an official of the same gender, split into two bottles and sealed by the rider.

● A code number's attached to the bottle and recorded on the relevant paperwork to ensure accuracy and anonymity.

● The athlete completes a medical declaration stating all medicines and drugs consumed in the past week. If any of these substances are on the WADA prohibited list, the athlete must hold a therapeutic use exemption (TUE).

● Both parties sign the form and each is given a copy.

● Both samples are sent to a WADA-accredited laboratory (if there's not one on site). Sample 'A' is tested using gas chromatography – which separates the contents of the sample – and mass spectrometry – which provides the molecular specification of the compounds. If the result is positive, the athlete is notified before sample 'B' is tested.

● The athlete or representative is allowed to be present at the unsealing and testing of the second sample. If this is positive, too, the relevant sporting organisation is notified and will decide on subsequent punishment.

 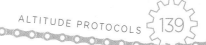

# Blood passport

○ The athletes' blood passport (ABP) been much trumpeted but how does it differ from existing testing methods? Over to Olivier Banuls, manager of the Cycling Anti-Doping Foundation (CADF), essentially the UCI's drug-testing arm.

'Tests cover a period of time and are examined for the effects of the substance abuse rather than focusing on the actual substance itself. It means we can analyse whether there are any anomalous fluctuations in any of the indirect markers of drug abuse.'

Whereas traditional tests look directly at, for example, the level and type of erythropoietin (EPO) in urine, the ABP analyses biological markers of doping. 'The reason is that the traditional approach has limitations when an athlete may be using substances on an intermittent or low-dose basis,' says Banuls. 'The ABP is more reliable.'

In theory, the measurements taken cover three 'modules': haematological (blood doping), steroid abuse and manipulation of the endocrine system (hormone abuse like human growth hormone). Since the ABP's launch in 2008, only the blood module had clear guidelines. WADA recently added the steroidal module. 'We also collect urine for variations in testosterone,' says Banuls, 'but guidelines for the hormonal module are ongoing.'

The ABP analyses blood and urine but it's blood that's assessed for the haematological module. Once the rider's blood is taken (see 'Testing procedure', page 139), the main points analysed are reticulocytes and haemoglobin. 'These are the most important ones we focus on in cycling,' says Banuls. 'Together they produce what's called an OFF-score, which is the ratio of the two numbers.'

They're important in cycling because, ultimately, you can deliver greater volumes of oxygen to working muscles if your blood is packed with reticulocytes and haemoglobin. Reticulocytes are immature or new red blood cells, which carry haemoglobin. Injecting yourself with EPO will stimulate your body to produce more blood cells, increasing the percentage of reticulocytes. The other primary method of doping – blood transfusion – requires removal of your blood before re-infusion. That initial drop screams at the body to compensate by making more red blood cells, again leading to a higher-than-normal percentage of reticulocytes. But this is where things become complicated and why the ABP is so effective. 'While reticulocytes skew upwards after immediate doping, when you re-infuse your blood [with the blood you stored in the fridge], your actual percentage of reticulocytes then drops because the "older" blood effectively dilutes the new blood,' says Professor Chris Cooper, the biochemist author of *Run, Swim, Throw, Cheat*. Haemoglobin, on the other hand, plummets when you first extract blood but increases on re-infusion.

Haematological scientists have observed that most people have reticulocyte percentages in their blood of between 0.5 and 1.5 per cent. Some are naturally higher or lower but it's the spikes or drops that the testers are eyeing. 'In the past it was far too easy to mask abuse. It's much more difficult now.'

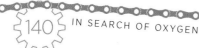

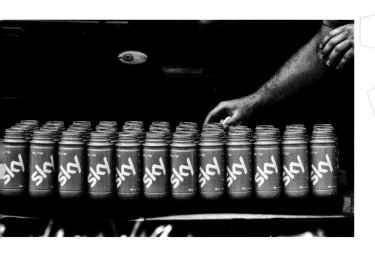

△ Keeping hydrated is key when training at altitude

metabolic shift toward carbohydrate utilisation over fat. (It also might explain why a 2013 study found that Americans living at sea level were up to five times more likely to be obese than those who live in high-altitude communities like Colorado.)

'Practically, it means you might have more pasta in your evening meal,' adds Pinotti. 'You also tend to drink more because of the increased respiratory rate. When you exhale you lose water. So increased breathing rate, increased loss of water. If you go over around 2,000m, you often wake in the middle of the night with a dry throat.'

That gasping for air is exacerbated if your iron stores are depleted. Iron is used to produce red blood cells, which helps store and carry oxygen. A low count means you'll be unable to create the blood needed to grab enough oxygen from the air and underperform.

'That's why when I'm at altitude, I'll usually take iron supplements and maybe a multivitamin,' says BMC Racing's Brent Bookwalter, 'though good nutrition helps. I have noticed that it's easier to lose weight at altitude. But it's always tough. That never changes. But I feel it's worth it.'

## CONFUSION OVER NATIVES

Good nutrition optimises the effects of all types of cycling, whether that's altitude training or in the weights room. That's an irrefutable fact. What's less certain is the effect altitude training has on riders born and raised at altitude. In March 2014, Team Sky announced that team member Sergio Henao had been removed from Team Sky's race schedule because of irregularities with his blood passport. 'In our latest monthly review, our experts had questions about Sergio's out-of-competition control tests at altitude – tests introduced this winter by the anti-doping authorities. We need to understand these readings better,' team manager Dave Brailsford said in a team press release.

'We contacted the relevant authorities – the UCI and CADF (Cycling Anti-Doping Foundation) – alerting them to these readings and asked whether they could give us any insights,' Brailsford added in the press statement. 'We've also taken Sergio out of our race programme while we get a better understanding of these profiles and his physiology. We want to do the right thing and we want to be fair. It's important not to jump to conclusions.'

When not racing around the globe, Henao lives in Riogengro, Columbia, a city located 2,125m above sea level. The anomalous results left Sky searching for the physiological adaptations that being raised at altitude has on the body. 'We are commissioning independent scientific research to better understand the effects of prolonged periods at altitude after returning from sea level, specifically on altitude natives,' Brailsford continued. 'Once we have completed our assessment, we'll decide on the right steps and give a full update.'

Henao underwent 10 weeks of independent testing in Columbia and at base level in Europe to determine a reason behind the values – although it's never been made public what the results were. The tests were carried out by a team from Sheffield University and the results passed onto the UCI (though the anticipated paper has still not been published). Come June 2014, Henao was back racing.

Like the results of the test, it was never made public what the exact anomalies were, though it would have involved his blood passport. The blood passport measures any significant skews in the production of reticulocytes (new blood cells), which could intimate EPO abuse, or old blood cells, which could suggest blood boosting.

Henao's case left many unanswered questions but one thing was clear: it showed just how much there is still to learn about the effects of altitude training, especially when it comes to nature versus nurture – a topic Dr Jon Baker, sports scientist of Team Dimension Data, is only too aware of.

'Something unique to our team at the [2015] Tour de France was that less than half the team were European,' Baker says. 'The remainder were Africans, and there was particular group who lived in Eritrea. It's unusual for East Africans to like cycling – more at home to running in the form of Ethiopians and Kenyans – but, like their running neighbours, they've physiologically adapted to altitude.'

It's a tale picked up on by Team Dimension Data's Natnael Berhane, the former African and Eritrean road-race champion who made history in 2014 when he became the first black African to win a professional cycling stage race in Europe, at the Tour of Turkey, and part of the MTN-Qhubeka team at the 2015 Tour.

'I was born and raised in Asmara, Eritrea, which is about 2,400m above sea level,' he says. 'My parents bought me a bike to get to and from school, which was about 6km away. I'd sprint against my friends a lot and it really built strength. I was soon racing a lot – around 35–45 races a year – and eventually made it to the professional ranks.'

Not only did Berhane and his fellow MTN Eritreans Merhawi Kudus and Daniel Teklehaimanot, who became a national hero when he wore the King of the Mountains jersey at the 2015 Tour, have the 'advantage' of a cycling culture instilled via Italian colonisation from the previous century and beyond, growing up at altitude gave them engines that, in the words of team principal Douglas Ryder, are 'at another level'.

That level is not yet matched with race experience and the demands of handling and tactics, but in theory, it provides a strong foundation on which to

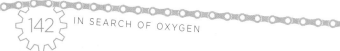

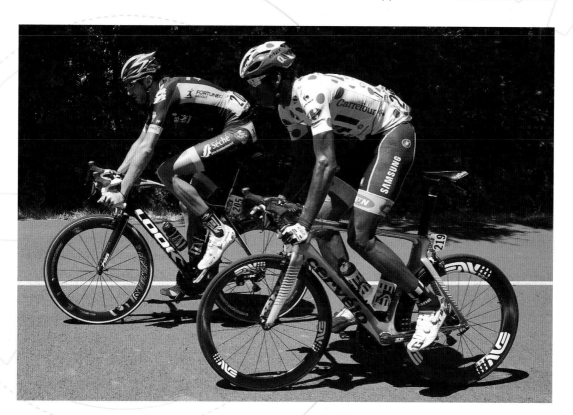

△ Eritrea's Daniel Teklehaimanot, wearing the best climber's polka dot jersey at the 2015 Tour de France

build future champions. Back to Baker. 'Let's take the European riders. Their haematocrit levels will nestle between 42 per cent and 48 per cent. From my experience, Eritreans are naturally around the 46 per cent to 54 per cent mark. Essentially they have better blood for being an endurance athlete.'

This has a knock-on effect when it comes to altitude training. 'For Europeans, sleeping at altitude means their haematocrit goes up slowly, let's say up to 47 … So those guys might potentially see a performance benefit. For the Eritreans it's a different story. They'll go to 1,800m and it's lower than what they're used to at home. So it has a negative effect because the altitude isn't as high as in Eritrea so there aren't huge gains to be made regarding blood factors. They also can't train as hard as they could at sea level so they don't enjoy a huge benefit either way.'

That's why Baker doesn't recommend altitude training to his Eritrean riders, despite a natural decline in haematocrit levels over time when living at sea level. 'It does drop but not to the level of Europeans,' he says. 'So for example, it might start at 50 and drop to 47. If they go back to live at altitude, it goes back to 50. A European might start at 42 at sea-level and when they go to altitude, it might go up to 47 or 48. Of course, there is a natural variation in the responses as well. You need to make an informed choice, and then test what happens with each individual. At the end of the day, performance isn't all about haematocrit. Recovery is likely worse at altitude, and unless you can descend to a low altitude to train, the quality of training is likely lower at altitude as well – you just can't push as many watts high up as you can low down so the training stimulus is less.'

In short, Baker suggests that training at altitude is a far more beneficial tool for European athletes who haven't experienced the numerous adaptations (see 'Altitude Adaptations' box on pages 132–3) enjoyed by athletes born and raised at altitude. Conversely, if you're born near the clouds but are then based in Europe, the higher intensity that you can train at sea level will outweigh altitude training camps because you're already adapted.

Again, this highlights the nature versus nurture argument. Are Columbians Carlos Bentancur, Rigoberto Urán and Nairo Quintana physiologically blessed for cycling because they've been born and raised at altitude, or is it simply the environment and culture that they grew up with which steered them to sporting success? Focus on 2014 Giro d'Italia champion Quintana and you're no nearer an answer.

'I come from a small village in Boyacá state that's 3,000m above sea level,' Quintana told reporters after his 2010 Tour de L'Avenir victory that brought him to the attention of the world. 'Every morning I rode to school down in the valley 16km away. In the evenings you had to climb back home again. I did the route with five friends. I was the strongest so I started racing. I did my first race aged 16 wearing football shorts and sneakers. That day I was bitten by the cycling bug.'

## SIMULATING ALTITUDE

Of course, in this ever-growing virtual world, there is another method of altitude training: live low/train high – in other words, the altitude tent. 'We've loaned out tents to many professionals,' says the Altitude Centre's Sam Rees, 'but issues of confidentiality mean we can't say to whom.' Some teams aren't quite as covert about their use. The old Slipstream-Chipotle jersey, for instance, used to feature the CAT logo, a manufacturer of altitude tents. Wiggins tweeted in 2012: 'Sleeping in my tent tonight after nearly a kilo of my wife's beetroot soup. You know what comes next.'

The revelation was hardly explosive – unlike the beetroot soup. Like altitude training, the theory is simple, if not slightly impractical. A tent placed over your bed uses what is essentially an adapted oxygen concentrator. These were developed for patients needing extra oxygen in the comfort of their home. Athletes use a generator that works in reverse, essentially sucking oxygen-rich air out of the tent and exhaling oxygen-depleted air into the tent – so mimicking the oxygen depleted air you'd be sleeping in at the top of a mountain, without having to leave your house.

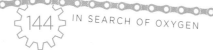

You can alter the settings to simulate the altitude you're looking to sleep at. For instance, 3,000m above sea level equates to an oxygen percentage of around 15 per cent. Their prevalence in the professional peloton suggests they elicit similar benefits to training camps, albeit in a more impractical manner.

'I've predominantly used altitude tents over training camps because I race so much,' says de Kort. 'I'd be home for 10 days and then maybe away for a week racing, so I had a tent installed at my home. I'm not sure about the physiological changes but I certainly felt stronger. When I try and hit form, I hit the altitude tent.'

Delve deeper, though, and de Kort reveals that it's far from a harmonious solution. 'I used to have a big tent that was the size of a small bedroom. I'd have a double bed in there and bedside tables. The problem is, your sleep can be disturbed. Firstly, the generator creates a gentle hum and a frequent whooshing sound as it breathes air into the tent. Also, you can have very strange dreams when sleeping at altitude and sometimes you wake gasping for air. I don't know if that's the dreams or lack of oxygen! I ended up buying a smaller tent.'

> ❝Sleeping in my tent tonight after nearly a kilo of my wife's beetroot soup. You know what comes next.❞
>
> **Bradley WIGGINS**

Altitude tents are a contentious issue, with WADA determining that they violate 'the spirit of the sport'. Still, they remain legal everywhere apart from Italy, who banned them in 2005. The IOC has also banned their use within the confines of Olympic villages since Sydney 2000.

Still, they look set to stay. Etixx–Quick-Step, home to Marcel Kittel and Niki Terpstra, spend a lot of time training at the Bakala Academy in Leuven, Belgium. It's a state-of-the art performance centre that not only has facilities to test aspect of rider performance like body composition and lactate threshold, but it also features a living room and bedrooms that are set to altitude as well. 'It's like a four-star hotel based at the top of a mountain,' says Etixx–Quick-Step nutritionist Peter Hespel.

Altitude training is a relatively new field that's being adapted and refined by professional teams all of the time. Many of Trek-Segafredo's team, for instance, went straight from an altitude camp in Sierra Nevada to the 2015 Tour, whereas some riders might not have been at altitude for four weeks by the time the race came around. 'It can be a bit of a lottery,' says David Bailey, sports scientist at BMC Racing. 'There's certainly a performance response at altitude but is that altitude or because the riders can focus on their training and recover better? That's why a lot of studies into altitude training don't provide definitive answers – it's hard to differentiate between altitude and focused training.'

It's clear that science still has some ground to cover before proving beyond doubt the empirical differences between altitude training and simply a focused block of training. Until then, the likes of Sky and Astana will continue to frequent the foyer of Tenerife's Parador Hotel.

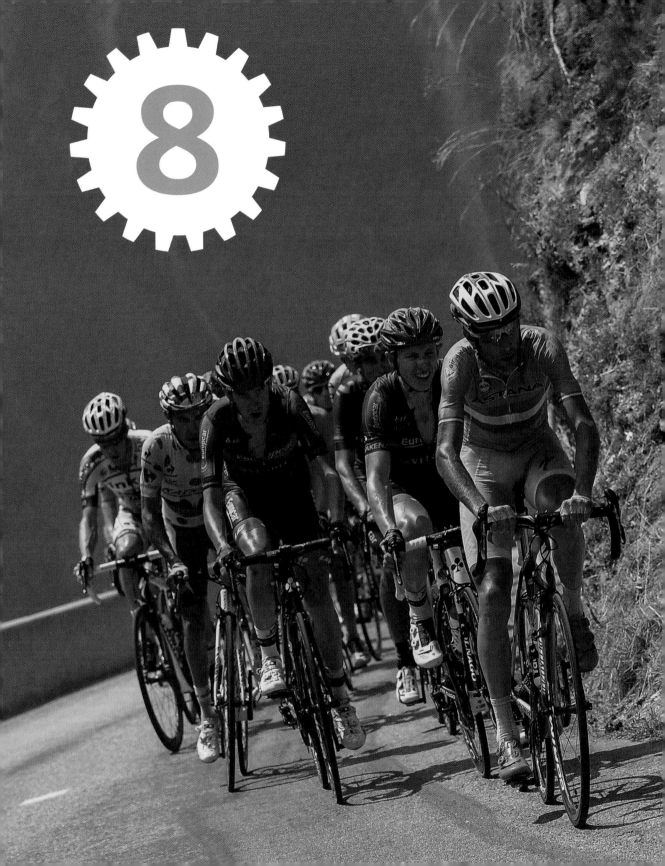

# PYRENEES AND ALPS

## ASCENDING TO THE GODS

**The first week of the Tour** de France could be viewed as a rather extreme warm-up for what follows in weeks two and three. Take the 2015 edition, for instance, which began with BMC Racing's Rohan Dennis winning the 13.8km prologue in Utrecht, Holland, navigated its way across northern France, before reaching the Channel at Brittany. Save for a couple of climbing stage finishes – the Mur de Huy (1.3km at 9.6 per cent) on stage three (won by Katusha's Joaquim Rodríguez) and the Côte de Mûr-de-Bretagne (2km at 6.9 per cent with stretches at 15 per cent) on stage eight (won by Ag2r La Mondiale's Alexis Vuillermoz) – the first nine stages were for the time-triallists and sprinters. At stage 10 it all changed. That's when the Pyrenees hove into view, raising a smile to the GC contenders and climbers – especially Team Sky's Chris Froome who flew to victory at La Pierre-Saint-Martin (for more on this victory, check out Chapter 1) while leaving Cavendish and Greipel pleading for flat terrain.

Beyond the panoramic shots of chateaux, the peloton winding its way past fields bursting with sunflowers and the aural delight of cowbells, the appeal of the Tour is plain and simple. Pain. And lots of it. And there's no greater generator of pain than the cols.

Take the Col du Galibier. At 17.5km long and an average gradient of 6.9 per cent, the Galibier was a particular favourite of Tour founder Henri Desgrange, who welcomed it into the race for the first time back in 1911. As the riders suffered with their leaden bikes and lack of gears, the poetic Desgrange wrote: 'Are these men

◁ Vincenzo Nibali, Cyril Gautier, Romain Sicard, and Joaquim Rodriguez tackle the nineteenth stage of the 2015 Tour de France between Saint-Jean-de-Maurienne and La Toussuire

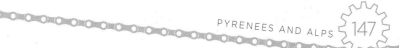

not winged, who today climbed to heights where even eagles don't go … they rose so high they seemed to dominate the world.' He also said that, rather less poetically, compared to the Galibier all other climbs were 'gnat's piss'.

# POWER-TO-WEIGHT RATIO

In 1998, the late Marco Pantani rode himself into Galibier folklore. With 4km to go, the Italian attacked with more ferocity than the torrential rain that provided an apocalyptic backdrop to Pantani's ascent to the gods. It sealed victory, Pantani adding the Tour title to that year's Giro d'Italia.

Key to Pantani's victory – aside from the cocktail of performance-enhancing drugs that was allegedly behind his high haematocrit level – and one of the most accurate determinants of how well a rider will climb, was his power-to-weight ratio. That differs to the flat stages, where absolute power – the maximum amount of power you can generate – is more important, as the muscular Andre Greipel can testify. The German can reportedly max out at a similar level to Marcel Kittel – around 1,900 watts. Because frontal area between a smaller and larger rider is relatively insignificant, the heavier sprinter can rely on that immense power to beat the competition. But when the terrain starts to rise, the riders face the ever-increasing challenge of gravity; in other words, Kittel's 82kg mass becomes harder to lug around. That's why, when the mountains come calling, the amount of power a rider can generate *in relation to their body weight* matters more than their maximum power output.

Let's use Kittel and noted climber Nairo Quintana as examples. Say Kittel's maximum power output is 450 watts and Quintana's is 360 watts. Clearly that's a significant difference. But Kittel's 82kg frame is also significantly heavier than Quintana's featherweight 58kg. To calculate each rider's power-to-weight ratio, you simply divide their maximum output by their weight. So in Kittel's case, his power-to-weight is 5.49 watts per kilogram (W/kg); Quintana, on the other hand, comes in at 6.21W/kg. Basically, when the gradient rises, Kittel's extra muscle mass becomes a hindrance rather than an advantage.

'I've discovered over the years that on the climbs it's vital that you can push a lot of watts per kilogram,' says Bauke Mollema, who's regarded as one of the finest climbers in the peloton. 'You have to be light but still be powerful. Some riders can push high watts but only for a short period of time, and not for the 30–60 minutes that you might need in the Pyrenees and Alps.'

So what is a good power-to-weight ratio? For the interests of comparison, and not to belittle the millions of recreational riders around the world, typical ratios are around 5.7–6W/kg for the pros, 3W/kg for keen recreational riders and less than 2W/kg for leisure riders.

Ross Tucker is an exercise physiologist from South Africa and runs the acclaimed sportsscientists.com website. Tucker has analysed numerous Tour

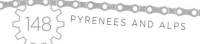

▽ Andre Greipel
and Marcel Kittel are
hampered by their
extra muscle mass
when the gradient
rises

performances over the years and calculated that the power output in the front group on ascents is around 6W/kg. During the era of discontent – where doping was rife – it was more like 6.4–6.7W/kg. This was reflected in the times. In 2001, Lance Armstrong stormed up Alpe d'Huez, the 13.8km-long iconic climb that features 21 hairpins and 'enjoys' an average gradient of 8.1 per cent, in 38 minutes 3 seconds; in 2011, stage winner Pierre Rolland took 41 minutes 57 seconds.

Tucker has plotted a graph showing the estimated power-to-weight ratio of the respective winners of the Tour during their final climb to victory between the years 1989 and 2004. When Greg LeMond won in 1989 and 1990, he hit 5.7. That dropped to around 5.3 for the first of Miguel Indurain's five titles in 1991, plum-meting to under five when the Spaniard won the following year. Then things climbed. And climbed …

In 1996, Bjarne Riis registered 6.47, Ullrich 6.33 in 1997 and a scarcely believable 6.63 when Pantani won in 1998. Then, the daddy of them all – Lance Armstrong's 6.97W/kg ascending Alpe d'Huez in 2004.

Modern riders like Froome, Nibali and Quintana are more around the 6W/kg mark, though power-to-weight does have its limitations. Team Sky's head of athlete performance Tim Kerrison explained to reporters that power-to-weight ratio isn't an absolute when it comes to predicting hill performance. 'There are many variables

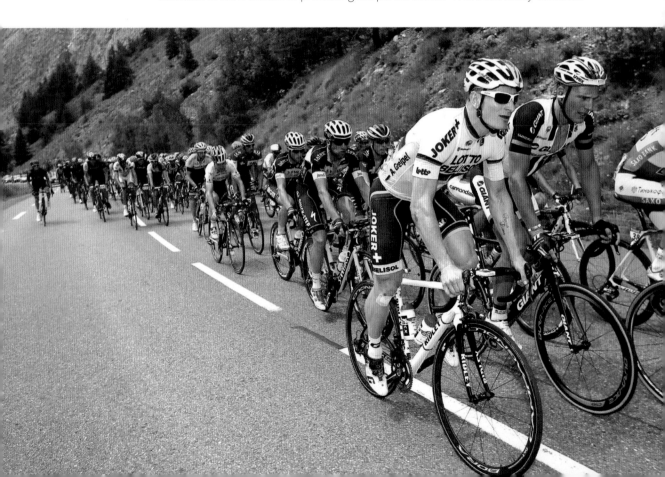

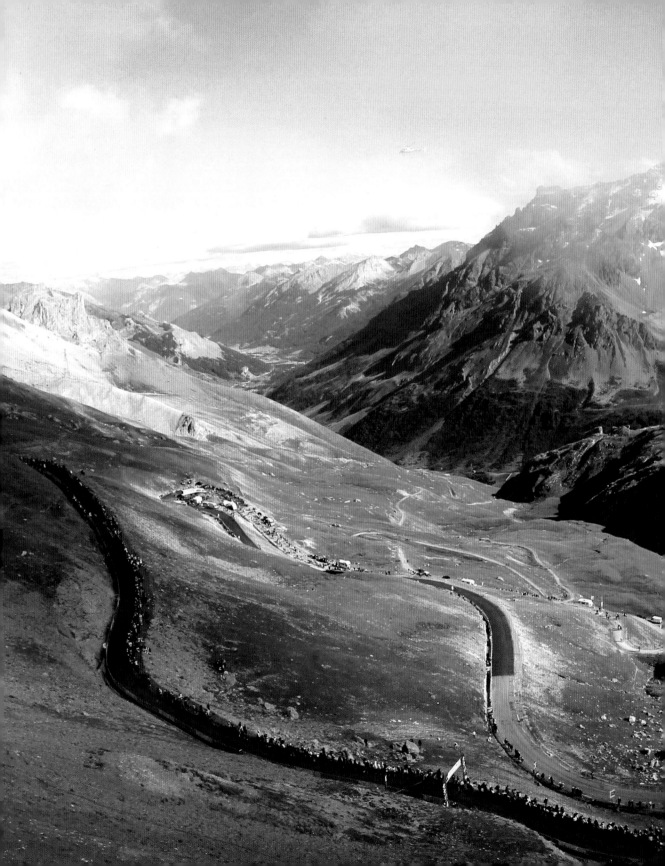

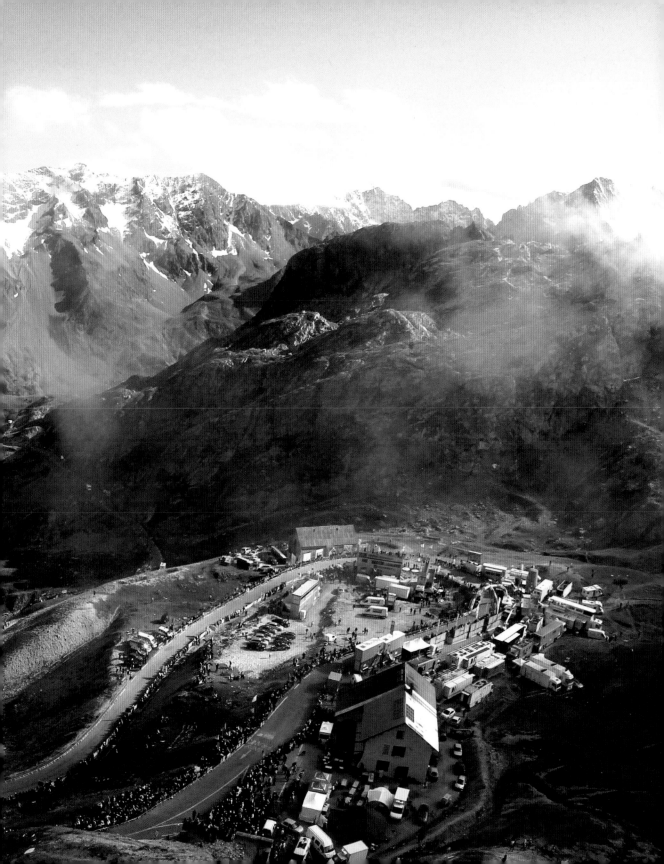

that affect it,' he said. 'They include the gradient of the climb, if they're climbing solo or in a group, the temperature and humidity, the wind direction, where that climb occurs in a race. And there's a big difference between a climb that goes from sea level to 1000m, versus one that starts at 1,000m and goes to 2,000m in the power the athlete can produce. It could be the exact same climb, but depending on the altitude the athlete will produce two very different power outputs.'

'That 6W/kg is a touch too broad when you're looking at a climber's potential,' adds former head of sport science at Tinkoff Sport, Daniel Healey. 'That number tends to be picked up by the media from a rider's functional threshold [the power output a rider can hold for one hour; see Chapter 1] but at Tinkoff Sport, we have numbers not just for your 30-minute, 40-minute and 60-minute efforts, which is kind of your long climbs, but figures from our riders for 1-minute to 5-minute bursts, up to 10 minutes, for shorter, more punchy climbs. Those figures are also useful when you're talking about sprinters. Of course, we won't publish the results of our riders – we don't want to give our competition an insight – but we have some

PREVIOUS PAGES
The Col du Galibier during stage 18 of the 2011 Tour de France between Pinerolo and Galibier Serre-Chevalier

▽ Lance Armstrong's power-to-weight ratio benefitted from nefarious means

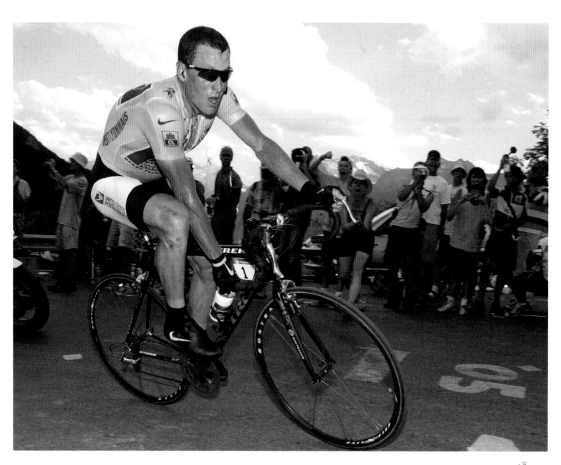

# Power-to-weight importance

○ Sports scientist Ross Tucker, who runs the respected sportsscientist.com website, charted the estimated power-to-weight ratios of the respective winners of the Tour during their final climb to victory between the years 1989 and 2004. Though not a 100 per cent conclusive factor in whether a rider doped or not, it's interesting to note that the highest figures were recorded by three confessed dopers (Lance Armstrong, Jan Ullrich and Bjarne Riis) and one who received a ban for high haematocrit levels and for whom question marks hung over his career (Marco Pantani). Miguel Indurain and Greg LeMond, with eight Tour titles between them, never tested positive for any illegal performance-enhancing drugs.

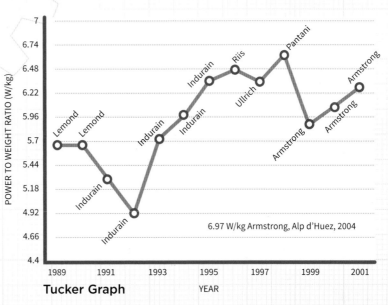

6.97 W/kg Armstrong, Alp d'Huez, 2004

**Tucker Graph**

key power-to-weight figures that result in strong outcomes over different types of climb. In short, 6W/kg is good for an hour but it's rubbish for one minute.'

In Hunter Allen and Dr Andrew Coggan's acclaimed book *Training and Racing with a Power Meter*, the authors and exercise physiologists include a comprehensive table of data that illustrates world-class power-to-weight ratio figures from 5-second bursts to an hour (functional threshold). For world-class men, functional threshold is given as 6.4W/kg. This figure increases to 7.6W/kg over 5 minutes, 11.5W/kg for 1 minute and 24.04W/kg for 5 seconds.

This changing of gears – physiological not mechanical – is vital during the Pyrenees and Alps, where the Tour can be won or lost in the matter of a few hundred metres. So it proved during the 2013 Tour on the slopes of Mont Ventoux, where a powerful and prolonged acceleration by Chris Froome left one of his most fearsome rivals, Alberto Contador, for dead. (Of course, Contador took revenge just over a year later at the Vuelta.)

# BUILD POWER OR REDUCE WEIGHT?

It seems a simplistic question but just how do the professional riders improve their power-to-weight ratio: do they aim for more power or look to carve kilograms off their anatomy?

'It's very strategic but also very simple,' explains Healey, whose disciples over the years have included Cadel Evans and Alberto Contador. 'You make them fit, then stronger and then more powerful. You can then look at reducing their weight.' It's a meticulous process that's based on sound principles of training and nutrition, tied in with the different periods of the year.

'Simplistically, we'd do general fitness stuff in the November and December training camps, before following that with a block of strength work in the New Year. That's generally low-cadence stuff. We'll then look to transform that strength into rapid application of force, which is power. We'll work on that up to and during the race season. But you definitely have to make the rider powerful first before you start losing weight.'

Each team will have their own protocol to help their riders lose weight but all of them will look to bring their riders' weight down in a slow and controlled manner. When Bradley Wiggins won his second and third Olympic track gold medals at Beijing 2008, he weighed 78kg. In the lead-up to his victorious 2012 Tour de France, he measured just 69kg. Nine kilograms is a lot but that's over a four-year timespan.

'We have a 10-week period where the riders will start weighing and measuring their food and logging the detail in a food diary,' Healey continues. 'So you look at the SRM data from an easy ride through to a moderately intense ride and then a very hard ride. You'll work out that the rider will use something like 2,000 calories for an easy ride, moving up to 3,500–4,500 calories for the harder ride and then 4,500 calories and above for very hard rides. Then you set up menus around that number for the guys seeking calorie debt.'

Healey uses some 'pretty smart nutrition' software that's available on the market to calculate a rough figure for food calorie intake – 'rough because the riders won't be expected to put down exact weights each and every time'.

On a training camp, where it's easier to monitor these protocols, the riders are then given a choice of three starters, three main courses and three desserts, all around the same calorie count – choice given so the riders don't feel entirely like automatons. The foods will contain the key macronutrients protein, carbohydrate and fat, with Sagan and his teammates served 2g per kilogram body weight of protein, which Healey cites as essential.

'I'll give you an example,' says Healey. 'It's not for a climber but weight loss is of a similar magnitude. We took a time-trial, rouleur-type rider down from 78kg in January 2015 to 72kg at the end of May. Now that's a big drop but key was that we conserved protein. If they're struggling, you can have big warning signs from the

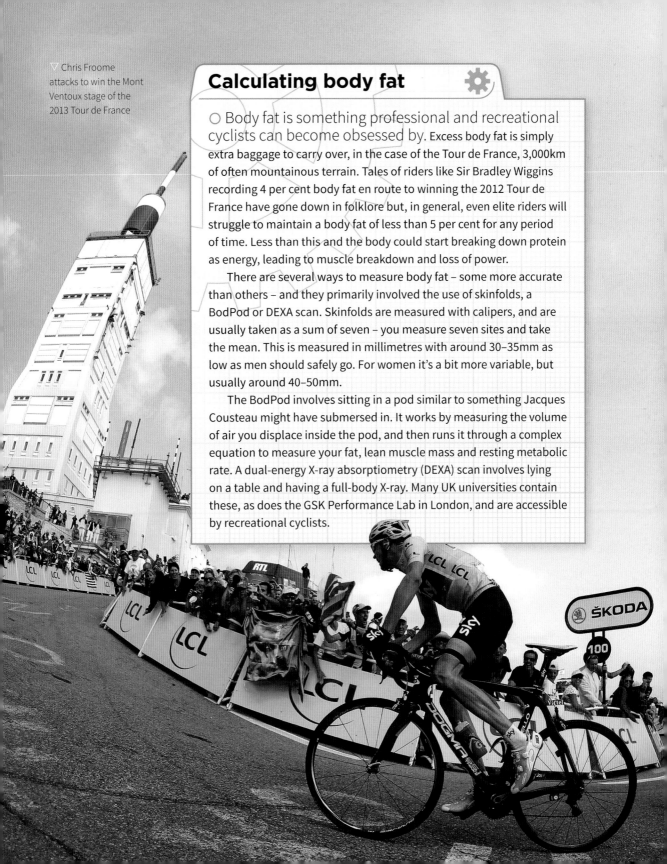

# Calculating body fat

○ Body fat is something professional and recreational cyclists can become obsessed by. Excess body fat is simply extra baggage to carry over, in the case of the Tour de France, 3,000km of often mountainous terrain. Tales of riders like Sir Bradley Wiggins recording 4 per cent body fat en route to winning the 2012 Tour de France have gone down in folklore but, in general, even elite riders will struggle to maintain a body fat of less than 5 per cent for any period of time. Less than this and the body could start breaking down protein as energy, leading to muscle breakdown and loss of power.

There are several ways to measure body fat – some more accurate than others – and they primarily involved the use of skinfolds, a BodPod or DEXA scan. Skinfolds are measured with calipers, and are usually taken as a sum of seven – you measure seven sites and take the mean. This is measured in millimetres with around 30–35mm as low as men should safely go. For women it's a bit more variable, but usually around 40–50mm.

The BodPod involves sitting in a pod similar to something Jacques Cousteau might have submersed in. It works by measuring the volume of air you displace inside the pod, and then runs it through a complex equation to measure your fat, lean muscle mass and resting metabolic rate. A dual-energy X-ray absorptiometry (DEXA) scan involves lying on a table and having a full-body X-ray. Many UK universities contain these, as does the GSK Performance Lab in London, and are accessible by recreational cyclists.

SRM. They won't be able to do certain reps at certain power outputs, and they'll be complaining of fatigue a little more than normal. The reason is often because their bodies are getting too few calories.'

The body primarily burns carbohydrates and/or fat for fuel. During extreme exercise and extended periods of calorie deficit, however, the body can begin to convert protein into glucose in a process called gluconeogenesis. 'It can happen at any time during a ride or any time during the day so the trick is to have small meals often,' says Healey. 'It's also why you need a high-protein content in recovery foods. There's no point being super-skinny with no muscle mass.'

## SHRINKING HUSHOVD'S RIDE TO GREEN

Get it right and the results can be impressive – and not just when you're hunting down yellow. On paper, stage five of the 2008 Tour de France seemed inauspicious, a flat 232km between Cholet and Chateauroux – one for the sprinters as the race wound its way south. As the finish line approached, Crédit-Agricole's Mark Renshaw led out one of the finest sprinters of his generation, Norway's Thur Hushovd, to what seemed an inevitable victory. But Hushovd failed to deliver a second stage win thanks to a then-little-known Brit by the name of Mark Cavendish. Cav undercut the big Norwegian to claim the first Tour stage win of his career.

While Hushovd's 2008 Tour palmarès nestled on one for the remainder of the race, Cavendish racked up another three victories. Hushovd even missed out on the sprinter's green jersey to Rabobank's Óscar Freire.

'Come the start of the next year [2009], it was pretty clear that Cav was the fastest sprinter in the world,' says Rob Child, nutrition biochemist at Team Dimension Data, who at the time worked for Cervélo TestTeam, the team that Hushovd had moved to during the 2008 off-season. Hushovd had won green in 2005 and the ambitious Child and Cervélo were intent on winning it back. 'Because of Cav's speed, we devised a strategy that moved away from simply going for wins on the flat stages,' adds Child. 'That plan involved helping Thor lose 3kg in the final few weeks before the 2009 Tour.'

Hushovd was regarded as a classics specialist where muscle mass is an advantage. Come the start of the 2009 Tour, his body fat hovered around 7–8 per cent. By the end of the 2009 edition, that figure nestled around the 6 per cent mark. 'That was due to losing some muscle mass as well,' says Child, 'but we'd accounted for that and it didn't affect his power. On the contrary, his power-to-weight ratio went up, which meant he could climb much more effectively in the mountains.'

Like Healey, Child had prescribed a negative calorie diet but high in protein. It allowed the Norwegian to rack up significantly more intermediate sprint points

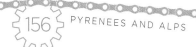

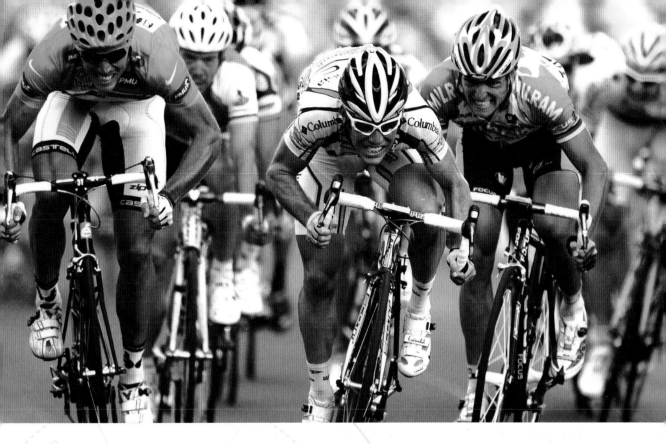

 △ Thur Hushovd
intentionally lost
weight during the
2009 Tour to win
the green jersey

than Cav. 'He lost every single final sprint to Cav [who won six stages that year] bar one. But with our weight-reduction tactics he won the green jersey.'

Child based his strategy on reducing Hushovd's body fat. Clearly the lighter you are, the faster you ascend but how low do Nairo Quintana and Andrew Talansky go before they either begin to lose power or become ill? 'There are a lot of assumptions you have to make to answer this,' says US cycle coach Joe Friel. 'The most important is what the athlete's power-to-weight ratio is at threshold, but without going through all of those assumptions, I'd estimate that a 1kg decrease in weight would result in a 1 per cent increase in speed. So for a 10-minute climb done at threshold, the time savings would be about 6 seconds with a 1kg loss of weight.'

Over an hour's climb, which many of the longer climbs are, that's a healthy 36 seconds saving from just a one-kilogram weight loss. It's that sort of statistic that convinced Sir Bradley Wiggins if he could lose weight from his track racing high of around 80kg, he'd be in contention at the Tour.

'You develop a lot of muscle mass, particularly on the upper body, while training for the track over the winter,' explained Team Sky's former sports scientist Matt Parker in 2009 after Wiggins had finished fourth at that year's Tour de France after dropping his weight to 72kg. Parker now works for English Rugby. 'We wanted him to lose that, but to do it slowly so that it didn't affect power,' Parker continued.

So weight matters, although Daniel Healey isn't a huge fan of gauging a cyclist's potential on body fat percentages. 'Skinfold and percent body fat is bullshit,' he says, not straddling any fence. Healey recalls how part of his masters qualification included six months focusing on anthropometry. 'It was basically hardcore statistics for six months and then you learn a process of anthropometry that gets you what's termed the ISAK qualification.' Otherwise known as the International Society for the Advancement of Kinanthropometry qualification. Catchy, eh?

'A proper skinfold process takes about an hour per person,' Healey continues. 'It's not just a quick pinch and you're done like too many do. That ISAK qualification taught you about the error in-between your own measurements; you learn about errors of two people testing the same sites over a certain amount of times; and then you spend the rest of your time using a statistics package to throw your errors out and get closer to the truth. It was like pulling out your teeth but it did show me that too much talk about body fat percentages from unqualified practitioners is utter bullshit.'

'The problem is,' he continues, 'I've been with riders who I've worked with briefly who are told they're 6.5 per cent body fat. The next time they're tested it's by someone else and they're 7.8 per cent. That rider's whole world comes crashing down and they set about losing weight. But those numbers were error-

▽ Bradley Wiggins lost 9kg between 2008 and 2012 on his path to Tour glory

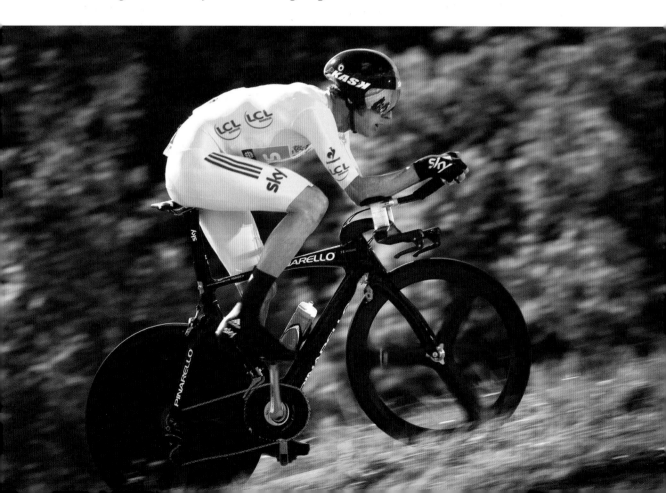

strewn, either due to the calipers, operator or even time of day it was taken.' Healey concedes that MRI scans get closer to the truth, 'but you can't have those at the back of the bus so they're not really practical'.

It raises the issue of inaccurate science resulting in potential eating disorders. An American study examined eating habits of international, university and club-level male cyclists in the US and found that 20 per cent were suspected to have disordered eating, based on their psychological screening results. It's an issue Healey's keen for his riders to avoid via constant dialogue.

'What I will do is show the riders the SRM [power meter] data and say we're here at the moment but if we get to there, and you'll tell me along the way how you're feeling, then you'll go this fast for less watts,' he says. 'That means you'll be this much further up the climb. If the rider is professional enough to accept a contract and also agreed that the team will help them become fitter, stronger and possibly more lean, via training and nutritional means [see Chapters 4 and 3 respectively], the rider must be accountable.'

# OPTIMUM CADENCE

Before Lance opened his heart to Oprah, the brash Texan proved as divisive with biomechanics as he did with the cycling community. While his main rival, Jan Ullrich, ascended in a high gear and low cadence [pedal revolution each minute], often settling around the 60rpm mark, Armstrong became famous for climbing in a low gear but generating over 90rpm, sometimes touching 100rpm. Chris Froome is also regarded as a high-cadence cyclist. When he blew his rivals apart in stage 10 of the 2015 Tour de France, ascending the 15.3km climb to La Pierre-Saint-Martin in 41 minutes 28 seconds, his average cadence registered 97rpm. This included a stage-winning 24-second attack where that figure rose to 102rpm.

Numerous lab- and field-based studies have attempted to unravel the mysteries of optimal climbing cadence with mixed results. Historically, 50–60rpm was the scientifically accepted norm but, more recently, researchers speculated that this low figure derived from lab tests of less than 10 minutes and at relatively low power outputs (lower than 125 watts). Instead, a study by Norwegian scientists Øivind Foss and Jostein Hallén tested elite cyclists to exhaustion using cadences of 60rpm, 80rpm, 100rpm and 120rpm. They discovered that performance peaked at 80rpm. 'I'm around the 80–90rpm mark,' says Trek-Segafredo's GC rider Bauke Mollema, 'though it depends on the severity of the climb, of course.'

A 2001 study by Dr Alejandro Lucia and his team at the University of Madrid monitored seven cyclists during Grand Tours and concluded that the preferred cadence during high mountains came in at 71rpm compared to 92rpm on long, flat road stages. Four years later, a further study tracked 10 professional riders during that year's Tour de France, monitoring their cadences over the different

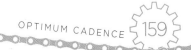

climbs: 73rpm for category-1 climbs and 70rpm for *hors catégorie* climbs (see the 'Categorising climbs' box, page 162). They also split the results into climbers and non-climbers, and showed that the specialist climbers spun their legs slightly more than the non-climbers.

Cadence choice can leave the most hardened sports scientist in a spin, but according to sports science professor at the University of Kent in England Louis Passfield, experienced cyclists have an innate preferred cadence: 'We tend to find most cyclists prefer their optimum and professionals know what that is,' says Passfield, who also worked with British Cycling for many years. 'From our research, you often see that their results marry favourably with laboratory results; in fact, in most studies looking at a cyclist's efficiency, we tend to allow riders to choose their own cadence and then hold it constantly.'

Norwegian researchers Ernst Hansen and Ann Ohnstad put it well when they said optimal cadence derives from an 'inherent hard-wired metronome' within the brain with this instinctive choice coming down to minimising cardiovascular stress or minimising leg muscle stress.

'That makes sense,' says Healey. 'If you have a rider who has a prevalence of slow-twitch muscle fibres and year on year they are used to pushing 70–80rpm on a climb, if you suddenly make them start pedalling at 90–95rpm, you burn out their fast-twitch muscle fibres and they fatigue for a different reason. So they're using a muscle group they're not used to and they fatigue fast. If someone's super-slow-twitch they're never going to have a huge cadence. Conversely, if they come from the track, they're probably used to high cadence so that works pretty well. And then you have the ones in-between. It's horses for courses.'

While the arguments are persuasive, some teams suggest that cadence of professional riders isn't purely dictated by natural selection and can evolve for the better. 'We made progress with Alejandro Valverde's cadence, increasing it from an average of 82rpm in 2012 to 86rpm in 2013 and 90–91 in 2014,' explains Mikel Zabala, sports scientist at Movistar. 'Our studies showed this resulted in greater efficiency and use of muscle glycogen needed for the final part of the stage, because low cadences require more muscle glycogen.'

Valverde's cadence transformation goes against the science that says the heavier and taller the rider, the more efficient it is to ride with a low cadence. This is purely down to the energy expenditure required to rotate the cranks – and the larger the limbs and the faster the rotation, the greater the cost to be paid. Valverde is no giant but in cycling terms at 5ft 10in he's tall enough to fit in the 'taller' bracket.

Ultimately, a greater impact on cadence boils down to the different categories of climb, which is discussed in more detail, in the 'Categorising climbs' box overleaf. Ultimately, different riders are suited to different mountains, and that partly comes back to muscle type. 'Muscle type makes a difference,' says David Bailey, sports scientist at BMC Racing. 'A guy who has a prevalence of fast-twitch muscle fibres

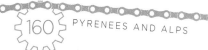

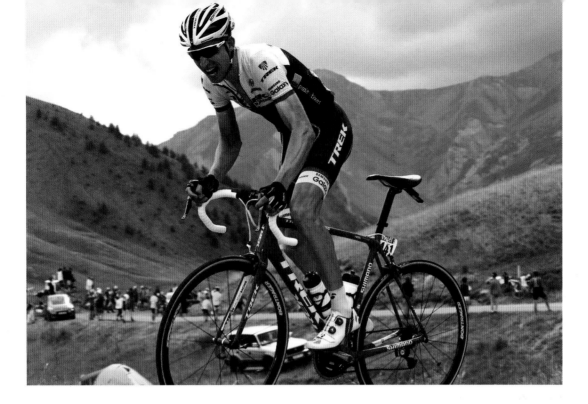

△ Bauke Mollema's high metabolism allows him to climb at high intensities

can generate high amounts of power in short periods of time, so might perceive the shorter, sharper climbs as more pleasant. Of course, these fibres fatigue faster but they'd have recovery time between climbs. A rider packed with slow-twitchers might "enjoy" the long, shallower climbs.'

'Nairo [Quintana] wouldn't attack on the flat or on a low-percentage ascent,' adds Mikel Zabala. 'The place he can inflict more damage is on big steep climbs, although sometimes in unexpected places.'

Without taking Contador, Quintana and Froome's muscle biopsy, you can only speculate what the ideal composition of slow-twitch to fast-twitch muscle fibres is for each climb. You can, however, be a touch more exact when it comes to fuelling your rides. The respiratory exchange ratio (RER) measures the ratio between carbon dioxide produced and oxygen consumed in one breath. With this ratio, you can calculate which fuel the body is burning to produce energy. An RER of 0.7 indicates that fat is the predominant source of fuel; 1.0 is carbohydrate.

'I've had tests on the bike that have shown my fat metabolism is quite high,' says Mollema. 'When riding, other riders started to burn carbohydrate for energy while I was still solely on fat.' In short, Mollema could cycle at a similarly high intensity to his contemporaries but fuel himself on fat over carbs. As a kilogram of fat contains 7,700kcals and the body can only store around 400g of carbohydrate (2,000 calories), the higher the intensity of exercise you can burn fat at the better, so you can preserve precious glycogen stores for sprints and breakaways.

'Out of the two profiles, I prefer the longer, shallower climb,' adds Mollema. Which makes sense as Mollema is still heavily metabolising fat at this lower-intensity but longer profile. It begs the question: can you manipulate your metabolism to burn more fat to help you climb? 'It's a hot topic at the moment, an example being glycogen-depleted sessions,' explains Bailey. It's a theme picked up by Matt Furber, senior sports scientist at the GSK Human Performance Lab, which has

## Categorising climbs

○ At the 2015 Tour de France, the race tackled the Col du Tourmalet, which has featured nearly every year since 1910. It measures 19.4km and has an average gradient of 7 per cent. At the 2015 edition it was deemed *hors catégorie*; the toughest category of climb at the Tour.

Most categories of climb are designated from category one (tough) to category four (easy). This is based on gradient, length of climb and crucially where exactly the climb sits in a stage – a 2,000m climb will feel significantly harder after five hours of riding than after one. A climb that's harder than category one is given that *hors catégorie* status. This term was originally used for mountain roads where

even cars weren't expected to pass.

There is no set formula for categorising climbs but, as a general rule, the following applies: *hors catégorie*, 1,500m and above; category one, 1,100–1,499m; category two, 600–1,099m; category three, 300–599m; and category four, 100–299m.

Legend has it that climb classification was originally calculated via a Citroën 2CV. If the old 35 horsepower car could make it up the climb in fourth gear, it was category four; third gear, category three and so on. If it couldn't make it up the climb, it was *hors catégorie*. I'm unsure of the science behind that story but it certainly makes a good tale.

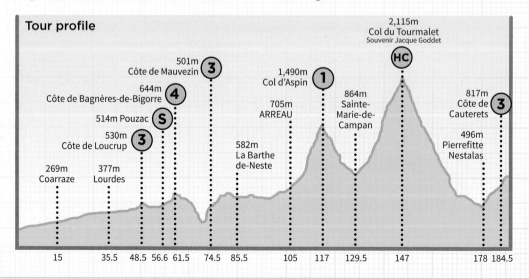

Tour profile

recently had Chris Froome through its doors for physiological testing. 'Theoretically, training fasted increases mitochondrial numbers. Mitochondria are responsible for metabolising fat,' he says. 'If you have, for instance, 20 mitochondria rather than 10, you can extract more oxygen, which you need to break down fats.'

Glycogen-depleted sessions and their potential impact on fat metabolism are discussed in more detail in Chapter 3. But suffice to say, it's just one aspect to conquering the hills. 'Tactics are key, too,' says Bailey. At stage four of the 2015 Giro d'Italia, Garmin-Cannondale's Davide Formolo attacked from the day's early break just before the foot of the final climb and followed it with a breakneck descent into the finish line to claim his first professional win. 'That was a cleverly designed stage because there were lots of shorter climbs so that favoured the early breakaway. You had some pure climbers in there, some rouleurs and a few others. Formolo then worked well during the flat sections with a group of around five; that number will work better at overcoming air resistance than a guy on his own so they could keep away. And then Formolo finished it off.'

Clever tactics also delivered the 2014 Tour de France King of the Mountains title to Tinkoff Sport's Rafał Majka. 'In the first week his instructions were to lose 10–15 minutes every day to the main pack during those early stages, so he could conserve energy for the mountains,' reveals Majka's teammate Michael Rogers. 'It worked because, as everyone saw, he was head and shoulders ahead of everyone else.'

# SEATED OR STANDING?

The sight of another Tinkoff rider, Alberto Contador, tapping his pedals, out of his saddle, as he conquers another mountain is an iconic image of 21st-century cycling. As is the slightly cruder style of Chris Froome, his chamois pad planted on his fi'zi:k saddle as he ascends at impressive speed.

In 2008, Professor Ernst Hansen looked at the issue of which is more efficient when climbing – seated or standing – and discovered that road cyclists were more efficient when remaining seated until the gradient hit 10 per cent. Then, with red blood cells requiring more oxygen, standing became more efficient. In fact, during all-out bursts of less than 30 seconds, peak power output has been measured at 25 per cent greater when standing compared to sitting. Of course, that's offset against the extra energy losses.

It's also been reported that even at shallower gradients of around 4 per cent, ascending at 19km/h requires 10 per cent less oxygen seated than completing the same distance at the same speed when standing. That's primarily because seated, submaximal uphill cycling sees the body's centre of mass supported by the saddle, thus conserving energy.

At the 2013 Vuelta, Chris Horner became the oldest winner of a Grand Tour. His 41 years dominated the headlines, but cycling aficionados were more concerned

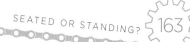

with his climbing style. 'I've never seen a rider spend so long out of the saddle, climbing in a big gear,' says sports scientist Louis Passfield. 'But clearly it worked.'

'When standing, the rider can produce greater leverage from the handlebars,' says former head of sports science at Tinkoff Sport Daniel Healey, 'and the wider the better to increase this lever. Horner at the Vuelta 2013 had super-wide bars.' 'Standing up also alters many of your body's angles with a key one being at the hip,' adds Passfield. 'By opening this up, you activate more muscles, including the glutes and more of the calves, which gives you more power potential. When seated, that "closed" hip angle can restrict power output.'

The range of hip motion from seated to standing rises from 42.8° to 68.8°. This is reflected in the knees, too, the angle opening from 28.7° to 73°. Finally, the ankle increases from a seated 25.7° to a standing 40.5°. 'These angles are close to what you get when running,' adds Passfield, 'which certainly pays off in the propulsive (down) phase.'

Studies show it's down to 'efficiency', which covers aspects like producing more power for less energy and how much heat you emit. Historically, it was thought that efficiency couldn't be trained but Passfield and his colleague, James Hopker, showed in the laboratory and out in the real world that it could. So when it comes to climbing, if you train on the climbs in the saddle most of the time, it becomes the most efficient style for you. It's the same when standing.

As heavier athletes enjoy greater support from the saddle than lighter riders, you could speculate that the 6ft-plus Froome has naturally steered himself into the optimum position; it's the same for lightweight Quintana, who spends significant chunks of time out of the saddle. As for mid-weight Contador, whose saddle often seems like sitting on hot coals, he's simply an anomaly according to Healey.

'Before I started working with Alberto, I used to think it was far more efficient to be in the saddle, but he's blown everything out the window,' he says. 'He just loves climbing like that. When you watch him, the central part of his body down to his hips swings from side to side. It's almost a little slinky movement that gives him that little extra push every time. And that goes against the grain, too. I always thought you should have a rock-solid core – no movement left and right – but I guess there may be some elastic benefits. Now I say, whichever mountain it is, just do what feels comfortable.'

The climbs of the Pyrenees and Alps are integral to the dramatic narrative that makes the Tour de France the world's most iconic race. Just look back to 1984. While all eyes focused on the duel between Bernard Hinault and Laurent Fignon on Alpe d'Huez, Luis Herrera fluttered away like a white dove. His victory was the first in the Tour by an amateur and a Columbian, and so well received was Herrera's triumph that the president phoned him that evening to send his nation's congratulations. The cols have proved a place of heartbreak, too, most tragically when Britain's Tom Simpson died ascending Mont Ventoux in 1967. It's that tightrope between triumph and tragedy that makes the mountains such an arresting part of the three-week race.

▷ Columbia's Luis Herrera used to float up climbs like a butterfly

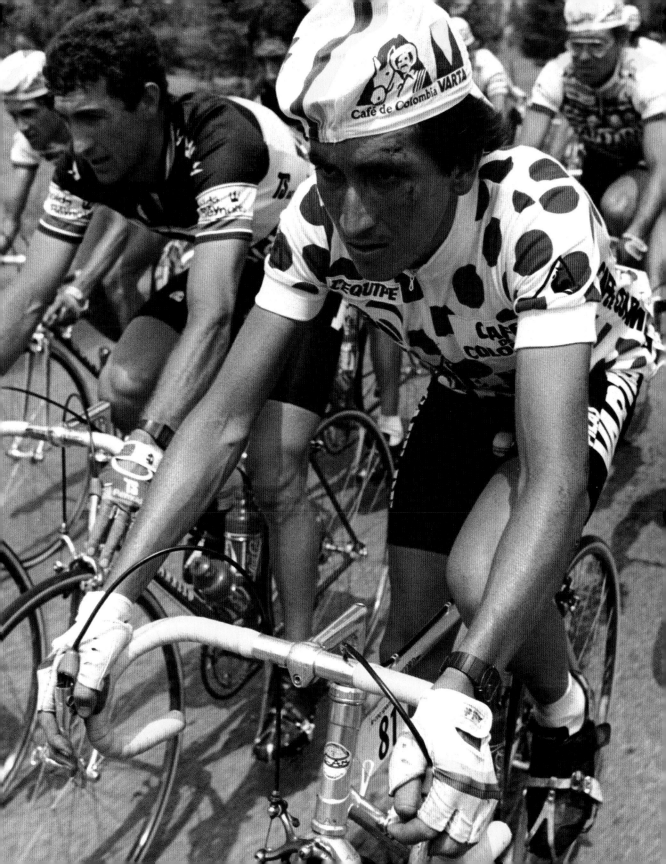

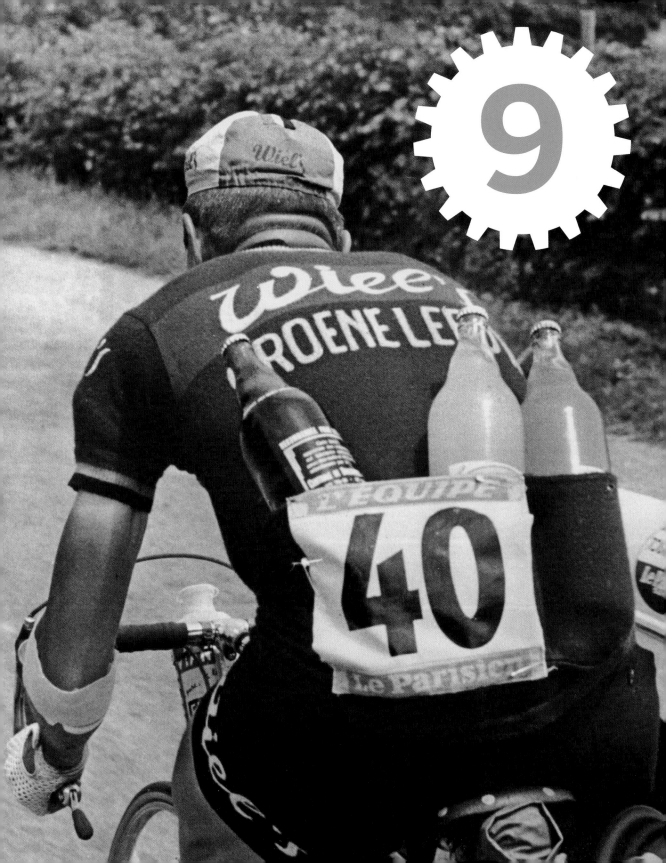

# RACE FUELLING

'The key over a three-week stage race is to pack in the calories. That means eating – and eating a lot – during breakfast, on the bike and dinner. Basically, eat until you can't eat much more.' That's the nutritional overview from Lotto-Soudal sprinter Greg Henderson, who's raced the Tour de France five times.

Fuelling such a monumental challenge has in the past seen riders eating steaks on their bikes and nibbling on baguettes. In the 1904 edition, the winner, France's Henri Cornet, reportedly fuelled on a daily diet that comprised 11 litres of hot chocolate, four litres of tea, champagne and 1.5kg of rice pudding. There was the curious case of England's Tom Simpson, who would regularly consume boiled cattle feed. The theory was that it would prevent stomach muscles from tensing up and using energy.

Simpson should have looked to the US instead of the local grazing field. In 1965 a team of researchers at the University of Florida created the world's first energy drink, featuring a mix of water, carbohydrates and electrolytes. It was created for the Florida Gators American football team and so was named Gatorade.

In the 1970s exercise physiologists began working with universities to develop exercise physiology laboratories, which would provide the ideal environment to study elite athletes. Come the 1980s, though late to the party compared to areas like coaching and exercise physiology, the field of sports nutrition had been officially born, with universities offering courses around the world and input into professional sport growing with each passing year.

The impact nutrition has had on the Tour de France is seen in the attrition rates from its inaugural edition in 1903. Between 1903 and 1914, just 31.1 per cent of riders completed the race. Come 1981 to 1990, this had risen to 72.2 per cent. That figure actually declined slightly between 1991 and 2000 to 67.8 per cent, though much of that was down to the expulsions from the 1998 Festina affair. Come the 2015 Tour de France, of the 198 riders who started in Utrecht, 160 finished. That's 81 per cent.

◁ Belgian racing cyclist Rene Van Meenen carrying refreshments during the 16th stage of the Tour de France between Grenoble and Val-d'Isere, 1963

 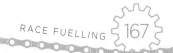

Of course, nutrition isn't the only reason attrition rates have dropped – training and tactics clearly play a role (See Chapter 4) – but the fact nearly all the teams racing the Tour de France now feature a nutritionist and team chef highlights the importance the team's general managers place on what goes into a rider's body. Which is quite a lot, according to BMC Racing's nutritionist Judith Haudum.

▽ Chris Froome eats as he rides during the 168.5km ninth stage of the 2013 Tour

## BALANCING CALORIES

'My primary goal is that the rider completes the Tour at the same weight they started,' she says. 'Yes, it's a difficult task but it can be done with correct fuelling before, during and after a stage.' (More on post-race nutrition and fatigue management in Chapter 10.)

Peter Hespel is professor of exercise physiology and nutrition at Leuven University in Belgium. He's also coach and nutritionist to Marcel Kittel's team Etixx–Quick-Step. He's covered countless episodes of the Tour de France and knows what a big ask Haudum's 'energy balance' intention is.

'On average, the riders burn about 6,500–6,750 calories per day,' says Hespel.

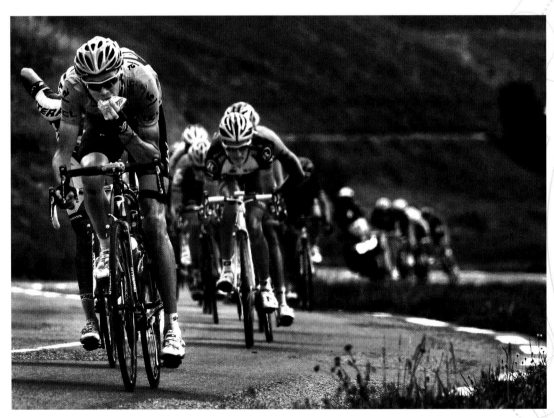

'Of course, that figure can vary significantly from day to day. A short time trial could be less than 1,000, whereas an exhaustive mountain stage that features five or six big climbs could require 8,500–9,000 calories, which is obviously extreme.'

That compares to Ironman (3.8km swim, 180km bike, 42.2km run) at around 9,000 calories; the Western States 100 ultra-run at 16,310 calories, based on an average 26.8-hour finish; and cross-country ski training of around 6,000 calories. All of those events, however, are run over a day or so. The Tour unfolds over three weeks. Take an average 6,000 calories a day over the 21 stages and that's a rather vast 126,000 calories.

'That daily calorie burn also varies depending on your role in the team,' Hespel continues. 'Every rider has a set job to do. You might have a rider going for GC who'll burn as few calories as possible by staying protected by his team and the peloton for most of the day. The lieutenants, as I call them, will expend the most amount of energy as they might be facing a headwind or chasing a breakaway.'

Hespel has calculated that during the biggest days, like stage 18 at the 2015 Tour de France that consumed 186.5km between Gap and Saint-Jean-de-Maurienne and featured seven categorised climbs, it's simply not possible to cover the 8,500 calories burnt. 'Even with the best strategy, that leaves a 1,240-calorie deficit.'

This can be overcome on the less-depleting stages, but the foundation for balancing energy demands begins with breakfast. BMC focus heavily on the carbo-hydrates and protein to pack the muscles with glycogen; jams, eggs and breads abound. 'We also offer wholegrain rice and pasta, though this might change to white rice and pasta during the final week when the riders' stomachs can find it harder to digest the fibre.'

Tinkoff Sport's Hannah Grant trained at the Fat Duck in England, under the auspices of molecular gastronomist Heston Blumenthal, and has worked at Copenhagen's renowned two-Michelin-star restaurant Noma. Grant is no ordinary cycling chef. 'I make my own breads, pasta … everything, really.' Grant's day begins at 5.30am where she'll begin cooking up each individual rider's demands for a 7.30–8am serving. 'We'll ask the riders what they'll want the night before. There'll always be an egg serving and however they want it – egg whites, poached, egg yolks – and we'll always use honey instead of sugar. Their sugar burning is extremely high so we complement the honey with slow-releasing carbohydrates in the form of gluten-free porridge. The oats are soaked overnight so they digest better, and I'll crank it up by adding nuts, seeds, dried fruits, cinnamon – whatever they fancy.'

Grant also whizzes up a daily smoothie, based on bananas and avocado, to get some calorie-dense nutrients into the rider. This is vital. Look at Hespel's calorie analysis in the 'Fuelling the Tour' box, page 170, and you'll see that deficit would have been even greater than 1,240 calories if not for a hefty 100 grams (900 calories) of fat. Grant's addition of avocado is a wise choice as it's a good source of good fats. 'Breakfast is finished off with my homemade Nutella with added dark chocolate

 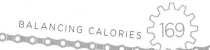

# Fuelling the Tour

○ Etixx–Quick-Step nutritionist and sports scientist Professor Peter Hespel analysed the calorie expenditure of a 70kg rider during a tough mountain stage of the Tour de France. The graphs show how the rider burned an incredible 8,500 calories. Despite consuming 12g of carbohydrate per kilogram of body weight (including the previous night's meal and that morning's breakfast), topping up with 90g of carbohydrate each hour on the bike and a significant amount of protein and fat, there was still an energy deficit of 1,240 calories.

It's interesting to note that the amount of energy derived from commercial products shifted from foods to fluids as the stage unfolded. This is predominantly down to

mountain stages beginning with long stretches of flat terrain, where it's physiologically and practically easier to consume foods. As the stage progresses and the mountains take over, drinking fluid energy is far easier. The team compensate this by consuming more calories than burnt over the less demanding stages, which burn around 6,000 calories.

| 70kg cyclist | 8,500 kcal | | |
|---|---|---|---|
| | | 1,240 kcal | Energy deficit |
| | | 900 kcal | 100g fat |
| | | 840 kcal | 3.0g protein/kg |
| | | 3,360 kcal | 12g carbohydrate/kg EVENING/MORNING |
| | | 2,160 kcal | 6 × 90g carbohydrate (540g) DURING RACE |

**Nutrition during the stage**

FLUID ENERGY

ENERGY FOODS

| 10–20g protein 5–10g fat | 10–20g protein 5–10g fat | 10–20g protein 5–10g fat | | |
|---|---|---|---|---|
| + 10–30g carbohydrate | + 10–30g carbohydrate | + 10–30g carbohydrate | + 10–30g carbohydrate | + 10–30g carbohydrate |
| 60g carbohydrate | 60g carbohydrate | 60g carbohydrate | 60g carbohydrate | 60g carbohydrate |

START ... FINISH

12:00   13:00   14:00   15:00   16:00   17:00

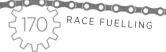

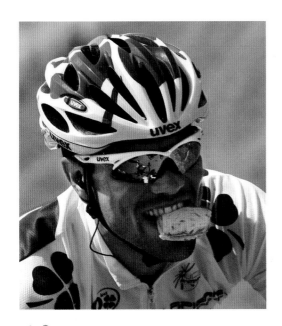

▽ France's Carlos Da Cruz eats a ham sandwich, mid race

and honey to sweeten things up,' says Grant.

The aim is to fuel the rider with up to 1,000 calories at breakfast. They might top that up with an energy bar – Tinkoff Sport are sponsored by organic nutrition company Probar – en route to the neutral zone and the obligatory espresso. And then it's all about on-the-bike fuelling.

During a stage, the meals on wheels comprise a cornucopia of energy gels, drinks and bars, all supplied by the team's nutrition sponsor. 'There are multiple aims and the strategy originates from the science,' says Hespel. 'The theory is that if you want to perform optimally in an endurance sport lasting more than three hours, you need to ingest 90g of carbohydrate per hour. It's from work done by Asker Jeukendrup and his time at Birmingham University.'

# 90G – THE HOLY GRAIL

In nutrition circles, Jeukendrup is Yoda-like. Prolific is an understatement with the Dutch professor having over 120 published journal articles to his name. But one of the most groundbreaking, the results of which changed the way many gel manufacturers formulated their products, was published during 2006 in his role as professor of exercise metabolism at the University of Birmingham, UK.

For years, sports scientists and, by virtue, cyclists were convinced that 60–70g of carbohydrates per hour was the most you could ingest, the reason being that transporters in the intestine (the group of proteins that facilitate the movement of sugars into the bloodstream) become saturated at that point and simply can't carry any more glucose into your system. But those scientists and manufacturers had made one fundamental error – their products comprised single sugar polymers like glucose or maltodextrin.

Jeukendrup had the idea of adding fructose to the glucose solution because fructose uses a different intestinal transporter than glucose. For reference, SGLT1 instead of GLUT5. Essentially, he turned the sugar transporter from a single carriageway into a dual carriageway. It worked.

Jeukendrup's results meant nutritionists could deliver up to 90g of carbohydrate an hour without causing gastro issues like sickness and diarrhoea, while the increased carbohydrate delivery brought with it more water so improved fluid delivery, too.

A further study by English Institute of Sport nutritionist Kevin Currell just a year later showed an improvement in endurance performance of 8 per cent when using glucose and fructose compared to glucose only. The reason is down to more readily accessible energy. Increase from 60g to 90g and you'll ingest an extra 120 calories over the glucose only option – 360 calories per hour against just 240 calories. Add that up over a six-hour stage and theoretically that's an extra 720 calories the likes of Nibali could consume without becoming bloated or nauseous.

Manufacturers like Etixx and Powerbar now incorporate this ratio of glucose to fructose in many of their products, though Hespel stresses that any more than 90g of carbohydrates each hour can have a detrimental impact on performance.

'I remember working with triathlete Marino Vanhoenacker,' says Hespel. Vanhoenacker used to hold the record for the fastest time ever at long-course triathlon, recording a staggering 7 hours, 45 minutes and 58 seconds at Ironman Austria in 2011. But that didn't help at all when a team of scientists working with Vanhoenacker before Hespel misapplied science. 'Marino was tested in the laboratory and the results showed that he could cope with ingesting 120g of carbohydrate per hour at race pace,' says Hespel. 'Unfortunately, come Ironman Hawaii, Marino didn't finish the run because of vomiting and diarrhoea. Problems arose because the test session lasted only three hours against temperatures that didn't eclipse 20°C. At Hawaii, you're racing up to eight hours in potentially 30°C heat.'

Vanhoenacker reverted to around 90g per hour and the issues disappeared. Of course, every one of us is different and, for some, 90g is still a step too far. Michael Rogers won stage 16 of the 2014 Tour de France. 'I always use a strong mix of maltodextrins and can squeeze some fructose sugars into that but it can be a struggle to consume 90g per hour, especially hour after hour,' he says.

BMC Racing's Brent Bookwalter says he's a 90-grammer, though agrees that like training your body to cope with the rigours of increased mileage and intensity, the same applies to your digestive system. Both have increased their ability to process food on the fly as the years have rolled by, though Movistar sports scientist and coach Mikel Zabala agrees with Rogers about the specificity of race nutrition.

'For me, 90g of carbohydrate per hour is too general a rule. You need to individualise. The way one cyclist uses fat or carbohydrates, or if he gains and loses muscle mass easily, or loses fat quickly, that can influence how much they should ingest each hour.'

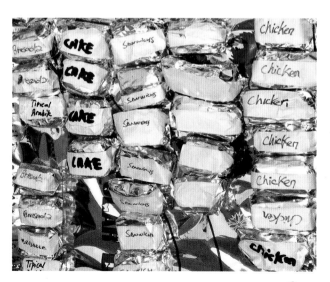

▽ Real food is a staple of every rider's on-the-fly diet

## Energy transporter

○ The illustration below might look a world away from the sunflowers and mountains of the Tour but it plays a significant role. It shows the absorption methods of different types of carbohydrate between the intestine and the bloodstream, which then carries the fuel to working muscles.

It's the work of Dr Asker Jeukendrup, who discovered that the rider can increase carbohydrate intake through a stage to 90g an hour (or 360 calories), from the previously accepted limit of 60g an hour, through multiple transporter systems, in this case glucose and fructose.

Delving deep into the science, the monosaccharides glucose and galactose are transported across the first of two intestinal membranes using a sodium-dependent glucose transporter SGLT1. It's believed that this transporter is full up and can't carry any more when glucose intake is around 60g per hour. Fructose uses a different transport system and is transported (independent of sodium) by GLUT5. All these monosaccharides are transported across the second membrane and into the circulation by GLUT2. As fructose absorption follows a completely different path to the glucose, it is not affected by the saturation of SGLT1.

The result? Froome and Contador can theoretically ride at a higher intensity for longer – vital for a mountain escape or tracking down their rivals.

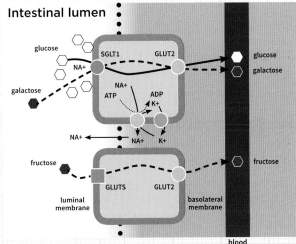

**Intestinal lumen**

glucose — SGLT1 — GLUT2 — glucose / galactose

galactose — NA+ / NA+ / ATP — ADP / K+

NA+ — NA+ — K+

fructose — GLUT5 — GLUT2 — fructose

luminal membrane — basolateral membrane

blood

# TIMING OF NUTRITION

Whether it's equipment, nutrition or training, bespoke will always beat a blanket approach. But whatever the sugar composition of energy products, their importance was underlined on stage 18 of the 2013 Tour de France. Team Sky's Chris Froome went into the 172.5km stage from Gap to Alpe d'Huez with a 4-minute-34-second lead over Saxo-Tinkoff's Alberto Contador. For 17 stages, the Brit had looked invincible. But now it was time to face one of the most iconic climbs in the Tour de France – Alpe d'Huez. The 13.8km climb, known for its 21 hairpin bends, had welcomed thousands of the sport's finest riders and spat them out with little regard. In 2013, the riders had to ascend it twice.

In the final 5km of the second climb to the Alpe d'Huez finish, Froome raised his hand and signalled for help. Teammate Richie Porte understood the call, and dropped back to the team car in search of gels. The diligent Porte soon caught up with his leader, who ripped the packet open … and extended his lead over Contador to 5 minutes 11 seconds. In fact, the lead would have been greater if not for a 20-second time penalty, the somewhat draconian rules stating that a rider may not accept food or drinks in the final 10km of a mountainous stage (20km for flat stages).

'I was really going into a bit of a sugar low and that really helped me with 5km to go,' Froome said at the time. 'It's a horrible feeling and I'm just happy to come out of it with more of an advantage than I went into the stage with.' And with that he went on to win the Tour.

Froome's last-ditch glucose hit shows the importance of the riders timing their race nutrition correctly – highlighted further by Froome admitting the 'low' derived from missing a planned feeding.

Teams like BMC Racing examine the profile of each stage, identifying not only sections that'll require more glycogen but also flat stretches where the rider can fuel more easily.

'We tend to front-load if it's a stage that includes mountains because they usually come halfway or even two-thirds into the stage,' explains BMC Racing's nutritionist Judith Haudum. 'So if it begins with 50–80km on the flat, we'd recommend an energy bar or two because they're easier to digest when the intensity is lower. We'd then recommend switching to gels and water, or gels and sports drink, as the mountains approach.'

Haudum notes that when the pace on the flat is higher, the bar of choice will be the Powerbar Energize, which is high in carbohydrate. If the pace is lower, they'll go for a bar that contains a hint of protein and fat for repair and low-intensity fuelling.

That template of low-intensity equals bar/high-intensity means gel is reflected throughout the peloton. 'If a mountain's coming up, I'd maybe have a gel with 20–30 minutes to go,' says Rogers. 'If you're hitting the last climbs with your legs packed with glycogen, that's a good place to be.'

Rogers suggests that Contador's a mightily efficient fat-burner, meaning he can spare those glycogen stores until he really needs them. It's potentially a factor why Contador's such a strong all-rounder – he has greater reserves to draw on when the intensity's cranked up.

As for how much riders will consume during a stage, Hespel's 1,240-calorie deficit model was based on the rider consuming what is deemed optimum, 90g an hour, for six hours. That's 540g of carbohydrates in a long stage, which based on

▷ Richie Porte's gel delivery service limited Chris Froome's bonking on Alpe d'Huez in 2013

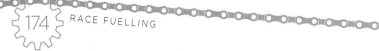

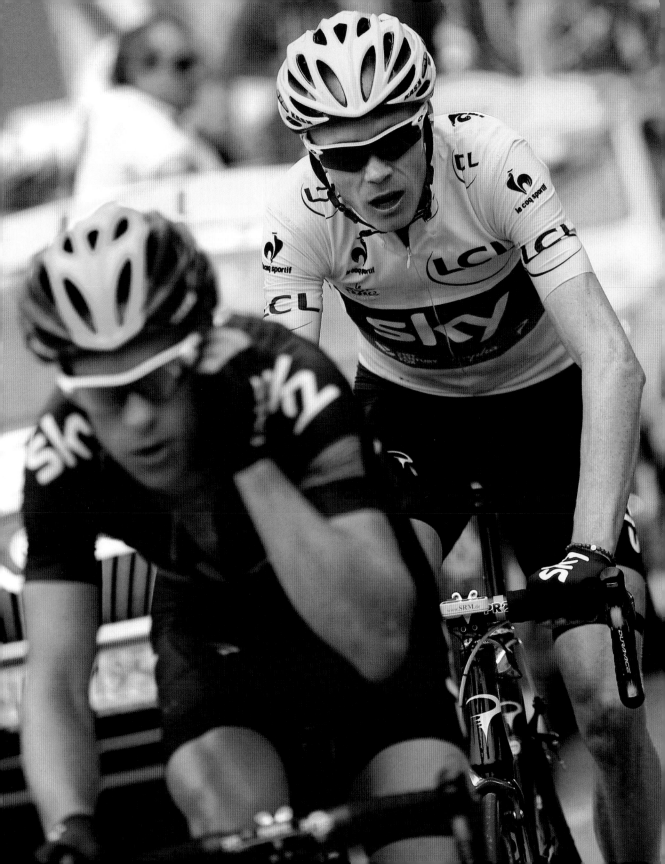

gels alone, generally in 30g packets, would equate to 18 packets. Eighteen sachets of sickly-sweet liquid, despite the mix of flavours offered by nutrition manufacturers, would quickly lead to flavour fatigue.

Enter real food. Today's riders, fuelled by a support staff that includes qualified dieticians, nutritionists and chefs, as we've already seen, choose from a race-fuelling menu that wasn't researched and designed in the labs.

'Most of our riders, including Joaquim [Rodríguez], have sandwiches with honey or ham during the race, and once they finish the stage, they tuck into jam tarts and rice cakes,' says Katusha's press officer, Paulo Grillandi. Etixx–Quick-Step's rising star Bob Jungels, who moved from Trek-Segafredo at the end of 2015, has a slightly more avant-garde palate. 'When racing I often have one with Philadelphia cheese, ham and strawberry jam.'

Twenty-two-year-old Jungels knows what he's doing. Ham provides protein and sodium. Cheese offers a protein hit, too. Chef Hannah Grant says her rice bars are a staple of the Tinkoff Sport on the bike nutrition plan. A further benefit of real food is that it'll often contain a higher moisture content than commercial bars, making it easier to chew, swallow and digest. Clearly that's even more important during hot stages.

▽ Bradley Wiggins (R) takes a feeding bottle from his teammate Mark Cavendish (L) during the tenth stage of the 2012 Tour de France starting in Macon and finishing in Bellegarde-sur-Valserine

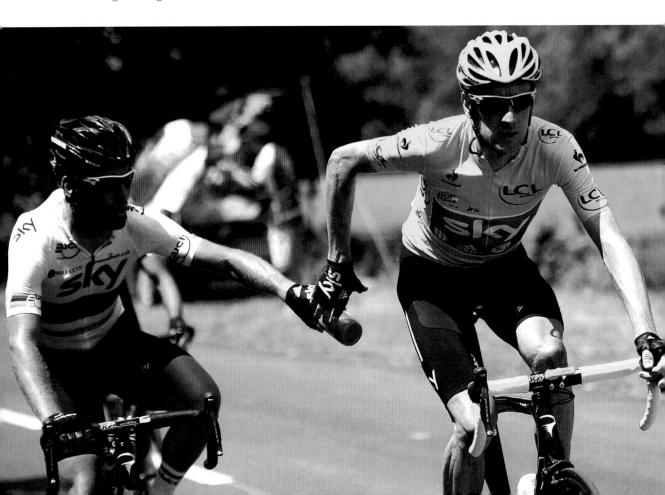

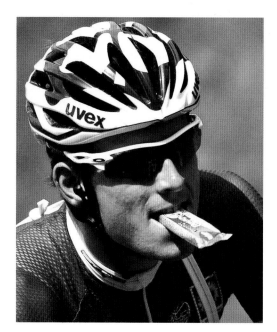

△ France's Arnaud Demare was saved from infamy by a caravan at the 2014 Tour

A mixture of gels, bars and real food is the ideal. But the physical stress of the Tour often leaves the riders' digestive systems in tatters – so much so that while you might think the riders would be dreaming of that next burger or burrito once they reach Paris, often it couldn't be further from the truth.

'My system takes an absolute battering at the Tour,' says BMC Racing's Brent Bookwalter. 'One of the things I look forward to most is not having to eat anything. The first few days after the race, I'll drink some coffee and let my body become really hungry and really thirsty. And slowly eat as and when.'

'The race becomes so mechanical,' he continues. 'You have to monitor how much you're putting into your mouth at all times. It's stressful on mind and body.'

That physical stress can reach a tipping point. At stage 14 of the 2014 Tour de France, FDJ's Arnaud Démare had to take an unscheduled pit stop in a spectator's caravan after a case of diarrhoea. Démare lost time, water and sodium, though retained his dignity, but it could have been avoided due to a growing body of research into the effect of swilling and spitting out carbohydrate drink instead of swallowing.

In a study led by England's Dr James Carter, cyclists were asked to undertake a 40km time trial. After a rest period, they were asked to repeat the test but this time they should rinse their mouth with a maltodextrin solution for five seconds without swallowing any of it. Remarkably, the cyclists were, on average, one minute faster with the carbohydrate solution.

Numerous studies have since corroborated Carter's results. Why is yet to be fully explained but there's a convincing case that the carbohydrate in the mouth rinse had connected with receptors in the mouth that signalled to the brain that food was imminent. This could potentially reduce the perception of effort, making the task easier and so the rider could go faster.

'This method of feeding would certainly have its limitations, though,' says Sophie Killer, performance nutritionist with the English Institute of Sport. 'Obviously the brain couldn't be tricked for the entire Tour!'

Killer suggests that this sensory activation could have played a part in Froome's Alpe d'Huez recovery, coming so close to the end of the stage. 'It certainly would have activated the sensors on his tongue,' says Killer, 'though a gel can get into the bloodstream in around 15 minutes. It was potentially the combination of the two.'

# CAFFEINE LOVE

▽ Peter Kennaugh of Sky Procycling enjoys an espresso ahead of stage one of the 2013 Tour de France, between Porto-Vecchio and Bastia

Killer's specialist area is actually caffeine – something professional riders have enjoyed a love affair with from the early days of the sport.

'Like most teams, we have an espresso machine on the bus,' says Trek-Segafredo's communications manager Tim Vanderjeugd. 'Most of the riders are big coffee drinkers and just help themselves. The machine empties very quickly, especially on the way to the start line. Sometimes it's the best coffee around. Hotel coffee isn't always pleasant to drink, except in Italy.'

Caffeine is a proven performance enhancer. The UCI, cycling's international governing body, once banned high doses of caffeine because of its perceived performance benefits, mental and physical. They rescinded that decision in 2004. 'That was down to caffeine's effects on an individual's metabolism,' says Killer. 'Caffeine's very hard to measure in the body because everyone metabolises caffeine at different rates. One rider could have a cup of coffee, then there may be no trace of it in four hours' time; another might still show traces in six hours.'

'Caffeine is so effective because you have caffeine receptors all over the body,' Killer continues, 'even in the brain. Caffeine can latch onto receptors, and each different area will have a different effect. That's why you have an improved cognitive effect that improves reaction time. In the muscle, it's a completely different response. Caffeine latches onto adenosine receptors in the muscle [which play a key role in energy production] that stimulates the muscle to generate higher forces.'

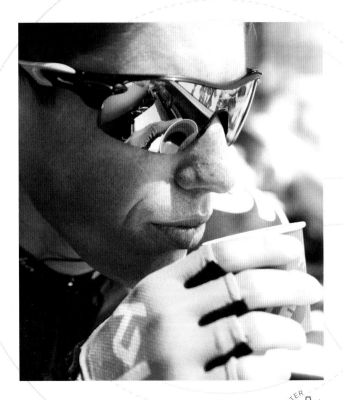

Caffeine acts on the central nervous system, too, to dampen the messages to the brain that the rider is getting tired, so it helps lower the perception of effort. 'Caffeine also stimulates energy production from fatty acids,' adds Movistar sports scientist Mikel Zabala.

How caffeine manages to do so is through being a master of disguise. In the brain, adenosine acts as an inhibitory neurotransmitter, meaning it promotes sleep and suppresses arousal. But when adenosine-lookalike caffeine is in town, nerve activity increases rather than slows down. The pituitary gland in the brain senses this neuron activity, perceives it as an emergency and so releases hormones that order the adrenal glands to produce adrenaline, which stimulates the fight or flight response of increased heart rate and blood pressure, which results in burning more fat for fuel.

How much caffeine the rider should consume depends on the desired effect. If it's muscular, like in preparation for a sprint, you'd need a significant amount, around 3–4mg caffeine per kilogram of body weight. That's around 200mg for a 60kg athlete. 'That's a lot more than you find in a gel [such as in Science in Sport's GO Plus Caffeine gel] but can easily be achieved through caffeine tablets or a coffee,' says Killer. 'One strategy is to have a strong coffee before the start and top up with caffeine in gels.'

'We'll examine the profile and distance of a stage and choose when to ingest something like a caffeine gel,' adds BMC nutritionist Haudum. 'If you have a mountain, like the Tourmalet or Galibier, you might have a caffeine gel so you're not bonking up the mountain. But if you want to be strong for the last third, you could take some halfway through and a little bit more later on.'

What's clear is that habitual caffeine consumers – those who drink several cups of cappuccino a day – are less sensitive to caffeine during a race so the majority of riders will abstain from caffeine in the build-up to an event like the Tour so they enjoy greater gains come the race. And when they do consume, it will be directed at targeted stages.

Typically, there are side effects. Caffeine's stimulant qualities accelerate heart rate, which isn't a serious issue but it can disrupt sleep patterns. That's where race strategy comes in. 'Lack of sleep is not ideal if you have a hard stage the next day so one option we use is to take caffeine the day before a rest day,' says Team Dimension Data's performance biochemist Rob Child. 'That way, if sleep is compromised, the riders can have a lie-in the next day.'

So caffeine is a proven ergogenic (performance enhancer) but not all riders are fans. Chris Froome has been quoted as saying he doesn't take caffeine pills on the bike. 'Instead, on mountain stages, I prepare my own bottle that contains two espressos and a lot of sugar and honey, which does me just fine. I usually have it toward the end of a stage,' he told the *Daily Mail* newspaper.

There has been controversy in the last few years about exactly what is going into some of the riders' (specifically finish) bottles though. Although entirely legal, these bottles are designed to stimulate a late-stage boost of speed. Often they'll include crushed-up caffeine pills and painkillers. Taylor Phinney cited that one of the painkillers commonly used was the opioid Tramadol to numb the pain of fatigue near the end of a stage. In Michael Barry's 2014 book, *Shadows on the Road*, the Canadian claims that he had 'frequently' seen Team Sky riders being given Tramadol in races.

It led Sky to release a statement, saying none of its current riders use Tramadol. 'None of our riders should ride whilst using Tramadol – that's the policy of this team. Team Sky do not give it to riders whilst racing or training, either as a pre-emptive

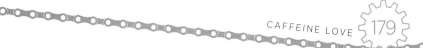

measure or to manage existing pain.' A team spokesman was unable to confirm the veracity of Barry's claims during the 2010 season. Allan Farrell, a full-time doctor with Team Sky since 2012, did tell *Cyclingnews* that Sky had used it but only as 'an effective painkiller when used in the clinically appropriate scenario. Certainly in our team we would have used it in the past but only when justified. We would have prescribed it, very minimally… sometimes if someone had an injury that justified pain killing medication'.

The situation seemingly became so prevalent in races that the MPCC (Movement for Credible Cycling), which includes Team Sky, committed to no longer using Tramadol during races.

And you can see why. Phinney described it as making you 'loopy', and in 2014, Lotto-Bellisol doctor Jan Mathieu suggested Tramadol could be contributing to crashes. Despite the anecdotal feedback, Tramadol is legal, though WADA (World Anti-Doping Agency) has put it on its monitored list. This is a bit of a grey area, the World Anti-Doping Code stating, 'WADA, in consultation with signatories and governments, shall establish a monitoring program regarding substances which are not on the prohibited list, but which WADA wishes to monitor in order to detect patterns of misuse in sport'. Caffeine's also on the list, which basically says you can consume a certain drug but not to such levels that it's detrimental to your health.

# BUFFERING LACTATE

Less contentious is the use of sodium bicarbonate. Its use as a sports supplement for high-intensity performance has been documented since the 1930s, and although it has never gained widespread popularity, it has been used since the 1980s in power events. Why? 'Essentially it allows you to produce more lactate during exercise,' explains Dr Jonathan Baker, sports scientist at Team Dimension Data. 'This means you can do more intense bouts of exercise, so essentially maintain a high power output for longer.'

Sodium bicarbonate – the fizzy white powder you bake cakes with – is what's called a buffer. When you exercise at an intense level, your body can't send enough oxygen to the working muscles to maintain power output. Your body is a clever vehicle, however, and can produce energy without the presence of oxygen (anaerobically) to make up the shortfall.

This happens in the muscle cell and a by-product of this anaerobic energy production is lactic acid, which brings with it hydrogen ions. The fitter you are, the longer you can generate energy this way, but even the fittest riders reach a point where the lactic acid they produce can no longer be broken down and recycled. That's when the lactic acid tips over from the muscle into the bloodstream, raising the acidity of the blood. Your body is finely balanced and the brain detects this unsettling acidic rise and then, through mechanisms which are still debated, tells

▷ The world's best constantly feed to stave off severe glycogen lows

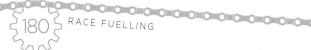

# Physiology of bonking

○ The bonk is a phenomenon known to cyclists of all abilities. Deriving from the original meaning to 'hit', the bonk refers to the catastrophic moment when the tank is suddenly empty; all energy is drained from your legs, they feel like jelly and, to continue the dessert metaphor, cycling becomes like riding through custard.

Simply put, your glycogen levels reach critical levels after being depleted through high-intensity exercise. Glycogen stores in the muscle and liver are around the 500g mark (2,000 calories) and if they run out, your body has no other choice but to burn fat instead.

But maintaining a high intensity of pedalling while burning fat is physiologically difficult because the body needs a huge amount of oxygen to break down fat. If supply can't keep up with demand, fatigue floods over the body, power drops and you feel awful. It's the body's rather dramatic way of telling you to slow down.

A cyclist's best protection against the bonk is to ensure glycogen levels are topped up before the ride via a diet high in carbohydrates, like pasta and potato, and then replenishing it on the bike through energy drinks, gels and bars.

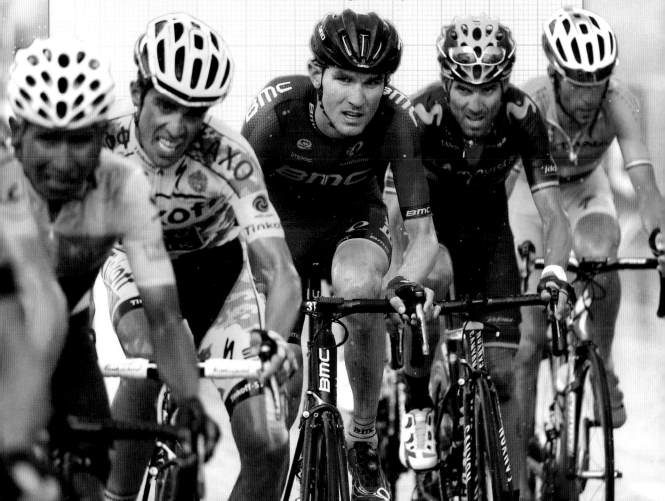

the muscle to stop working so hard. Power output falls and with it chances of *le maillot jaune.*

That's where sodium bicarbonate comes in. Because it's an alkaline, it neutralises the acidic threat from intense exercise and, in theory, means the rider can work harder for longer.

Numerous studies have supported the use of sodium bicarbonate in the professional rider's armoury. Research carried out in 2013 by the Institute of Human Movement Studies in Zurich saw Swiss scientists give eight cyclists and triathletes either a placebo or 0.3g of bicarbonate per kilogram of body weight 90 minutes before a critical power test – essentially the maximum average power you can maintain over a set time. That placebo or bicarbonate ingestion pattern was repeated for five consecutive days.

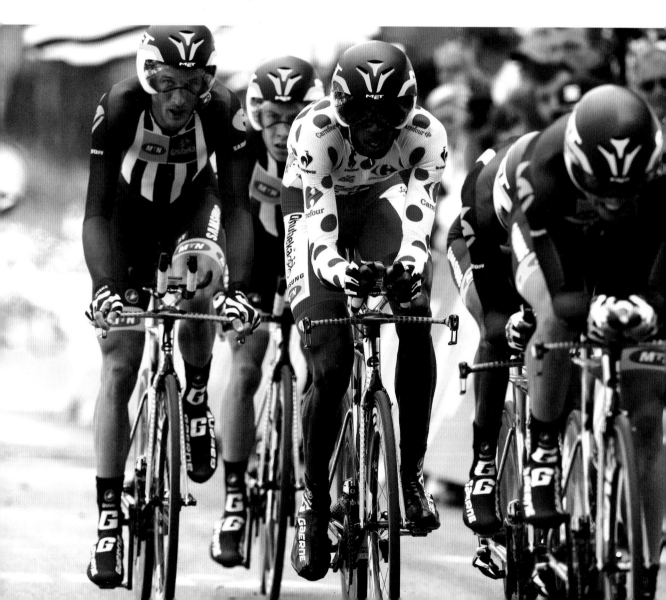

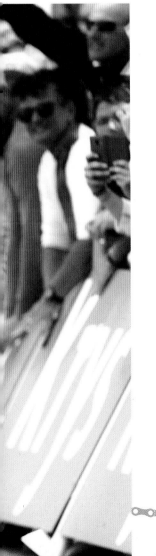

▽ Sodium-bicarb ingestion is a common nutrition strategy during time trials, as used by teams like Team Dimension Data

The scientists discovered that bicarbonate supplementation increased critical power output by a staggering 23.5 per cent, from an average 669 seconds to 826.5 seconds. This was maintained each day, suggesting that bicarbonate ingestion is not only good for a one-off intense effort like a time trial but for multi-stage races, too. There are potential downsides, however, including gastric distress and nausea.

'Many of our riders would certainly use it for something like the prologue at the Tour, which can be over in 20 minutes,' says Baker. 'However, how much they'd take will be determined through trial and error in training. You can do acute interventions. For example, in training we might give a rider 0.6g of bicarbonate per kilogram in water and ask them to drink it an hour before they race. That gives it time to enter the bloodstream. However, it's very salty and can actually make riders retch. So the riders can take it in capsule form instead. The downside is you'll be taking 10–20 small capsules, but it's still better than drinking it down.'

You can also take it chronically, where you ingest less for a longer period, so are slowly increasing levels in the blood. 'But that'd be no good in the Tour time trial, apart from the prologue,' adds Baker. 'You'd have used it all up in stage one, so acute is probably better.'

Baker also highlights a practical issue of applying research that worked in laboratories. 'There are around 10,000 sports-science journal articles published globally each year,' explains Baker. 'Some are high-end medical ones like the functioning of cardiac muscle in the heart, while some are as simple as an energy drink is better than water. It's our job to pick the best and most applicable bits, sometimes modifying the practice to ensure that what happens in the controlled world of a laboratory can be assimilated to the real world.

'That's why we often use sodium bicarbonate over sodium citrate,' he adds. 'There's research to suggest citrate's actually a better buffering agent but you can't buy it down your local supermarket.' Of course, a well-funded team could buy a chemist's worth of sodium citrate, but with riders racing and training all over the world, often in splintered groups of three or four – like specific training camps for the climbers in a team, for example – having a supplement within easy purchase is the ideal.

That's the beauty of working with WorldTour teams. Results emanating from laboratories can give some startling results, but apply them to the less-controlled and frantic world of professional cycling and they don't always have positive results. The next 'big thing' will come and go but you can be assured that caffeine, energy products and the humble rice cake will continue fuelling riders to the finish line for many years to come. But the feeding strategy doesn't stop there. Once the riders roll down the finish chute, their first thought is to begin recovery for the next day's stage. As you'll discover in the next chapter, that comes down to a mobile kitchen, tights and sleep – lots of sleep.

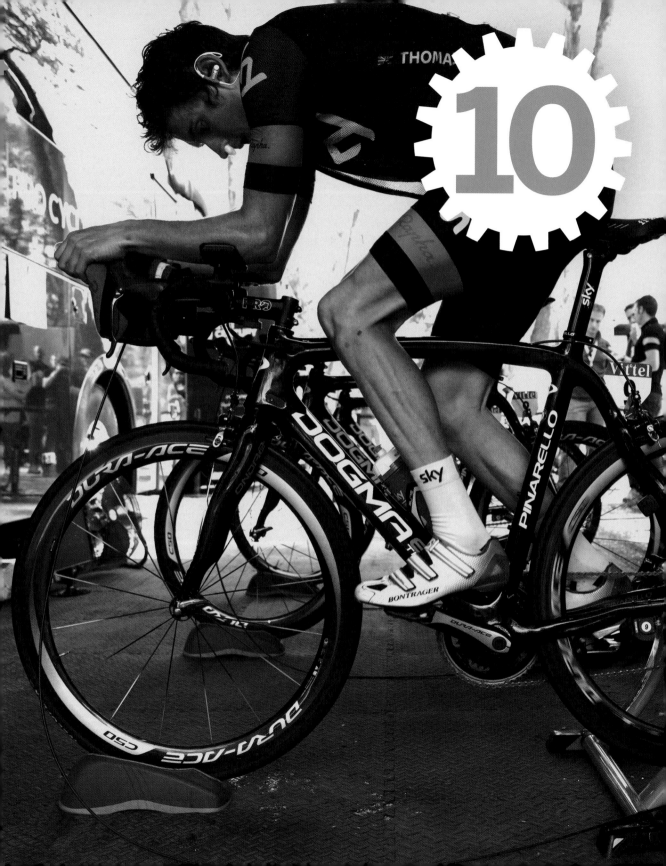

10

# RAPID RECOVERY

**The Tour de France takes place over 23 days** and 21 stages. Over the course of 2,000-plus miles, the 198 riders will be racing for anywhere between 84 hours, 46 minutes and 14 seconds – Chris Froome's race-winning time in 2015 – to FDJ's Sébastian Chavanel's 89 hours, 43 minutes and 13 seconds, giving him the honour of the *lanterne rouge* for last finisher at the Tour. For both riders, that's nearly four whole days of solid racing. That's immense, but calculated over 23 days – which includes two rest days – that leaves nearly 19 days and nights when the riders aren't racing. What are they doing with themselves? And what do they get up to during those periods? Simple – recovery.

'There are four things you do at the Tour de France,' says Brent Bookwalter, multiple Tour de France finisher and BMC Racing stalwart who finished third overall at the 2015 Tour of Utah, 'namely eat, sleep, transfer and race. Three of those are predominantly about recovery.'

With the use of diligent protocols and innovative strategies, the aim is to maintain power output from stage one to the final mountainous effort in the Alps. In practice, it's a difficult task. 'I'd have to go over my power files to give an exact file number but there's always some form of drop-off,' says Tinkoff Sport's Michael Rogers. 'I find if I can, say, maintain 380–400 watts for an hour at the start of the Tour, by the end I can hold it for half an hour. So you can hold it but for much shorter.'

The aim of recovery is essentially about keeping those power losses to a minimum. And the first step toward repairing the rider before the following day's stage begins the moment the rider crosses the line?

That's not technically correct, according to BMC's sports scientist David Bailey, when I spoke to him during Paris–Nice 2015. 'Only today I'm filling out the information from Judith [Haudum, BMC nutritionist] for tomorrow's stage [Paris–Nice], though we're also thinking about the final stage [the following day]. In particular, we're looking at Tejay's [van Garderen] strategy for the time trial from Nice to

◁ Team Sky brought the concept of post-stage active recovery into the peloton

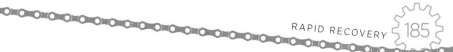

Col d'Éze. The debate is, if he does everything properly and recovers well, there might be no need to compromise bike and rider weight on that short (9.6km) stage by carrying a bottle.'

It's becoming more common that Tour riders will actually be recovering during the stage with a hint of protein in many of their bars, gels and drinks to begin the process of muscle repair *while they're still riding*. Admittedly, your body's energies are predominantly focused elsewhere – like fuelling speeds of up to 50mph – so the focused recovery really begins in earnest when the rider crosses the line – though before they've dismounted.

One of the innovations Team Sky brought to the peloton was a warm-down zone to run alongside their post-race media zone. Cycling is a sport steeped in history and traditions – 'manacled' by it according to Chris Boardman. When Sky riders rode straight onto a static turbo trainer after six hours of riding and began 'cooling down', other teams looked on with bemusement.

'I remember one of the first races I competed in for Sky was at the 2012 Vuelta Ciclista al País Vasco [the Tour of the Basque Country],' says Sky's Luke Rowe. 'We finished the race and hopped onto the turbos. The other guys were passing us and laughing their heads off. Those same guys are now doing exactly what we do.'

The idea was hardly groundbreaking but the application in cycling was. The basic aim of a cool-down is to return the rider's body to its recovered pre-stage state. A progressive cool-down on the turbo trainer of around 10 minutes helps to remove metabolic waste products from the working muscles simply by maintaining a reasonable blood flow around the body. Stop dead and head straight to the bus and the waste products simply sit in the muscle and inhibit the recovery process. So important is the cool-down to athletes that riders don't have to report to post-stage doping control until they've completed their turbo-training session. Not everyone hits the turbo, of course. If a rider's

▷ Warming down on turbo trainers eases out free radicals from the day's exertions

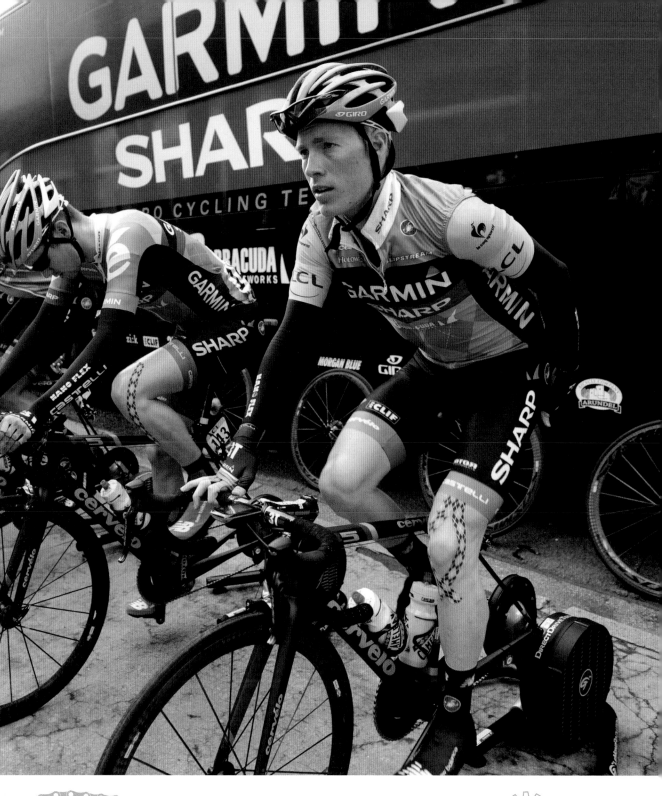

## Protein – king of recovery

○ Proteins are a chain or several chains of amino acids. These are the building blocks of life and perform a huge number of functions.

Proteins send signals around the body in the form of hormones like insulin; they form enzymes that digest food; and they play a structural role in hair, skin and muscles.

It's that last one that's of particular importance to the cyclist and specifically relating to an amino acid called leucine. Leucine's not only a building block of muscle but is also associated with the stimulation of muscle protein synthesis. In other words, it tells the muscle to begin manufacturing proteins to repair and rebuild the muscle. Whey and casein proteins, which both come from cow's milk, are rich sources of leucine so recommended for all cyclists, though be aware of their different properties.

'The absorption rate of whey and casein varies,' says Judith Haudum, nutritionist at BMC Racing. 'If you're looking for rapid absorption, like after exercise, go for whey. During the day or night, we go for casein because it digests slower.'

While leucine plays a significant role, however, Haudum warns that an athlete should be looking for the full complement of amino acids for perfect working function and, again, that comes down to correct food choices.

Tuna is a common food of the recovery Tour rider with 26g of protein per 100g serving. Further protein-rich foods include turkey and chicken breasts (30g per 100g), lean beef (36g) and pork chops with the fat removed (25g).

had an easy stage – it's all relative – and they've sat in the pack all day, they might head straight to the bus. But whether you turbo or not, all riders begin refuelling from the moment they cross the line …

## THE RECOVERY DRINK

'The first step in the refuelling plan involves a recovery shake containing a mix of carbohydrates and protein,' explains Haudum. Historically, it was all about carbohydrates as proteins were thought to come into their own only when repairing muscles from weight-training sessions. However, studies in the late 1990s not only showed the damage cycling can do to the muscle – especially when sprinting and climbing – but that carbohydrates combined with protein filled up the body's glycogen stores much quicker.

A review of studies into protein needs post-exercise by researchers at McMasters University in Canada concluded that consuming four-parts carbohydrate to one-part protein provided optimum speed of recovery, while another from

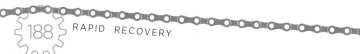

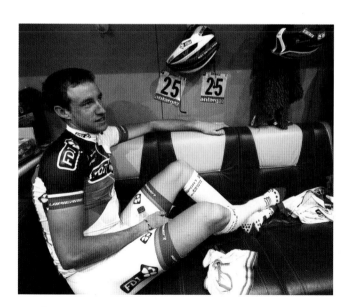

▽ FDJ are just one team who recover via compression socks

Texas University in 2004 discovered that a carbohydrate-protein drink increased glycogen storage by 38 per cent compared with a glycogen-only drink.

Just why the addition of protein is so effective has to do with insulin, the hormone whose main job is to transport glucose and amino acids to the liver and the muscles. The more insulin that is present in the bloodstream, the more glucose and amino acids can be carried to working muscles – thereby promoting glycogen and protein manufacture. Insulin also counters the effects of the hormone cortisol. Cortisol is a steroid hormone that's elevated during periods of intense exercise. This can lead to a phenomenon known as proteolysis (protein breakdown), which can result in muscle wastage. Studies show that when protein is consumed with carbohydrate, the insulin response can nearly double that invoked by carbs alone, reducing cortisol levels and accelerating recovery time

It's not just the composition of a recovery drink that's important – timing is key, too, according to Haudum. 'Enzymes and transporters are upregulated [increase in the number of receptors on target cells] after exercise, which means there's an increased rate of glycogen and protein synthesis. So if you miss out on consuming the right nutrition in the first 2 hours after exercise, you only take up 50 per cent of what's possible than starting straight over. So it might take 40 hours to recover instead of 24 hours.'

While the riders are sipping their recovery drink, it's common for them to unclip their bike shoes and slip into a pair of compression socks. Like many performance interventions that have permeated professional cycling, compression socks started out in the medical sector. Unlike EPO, human growth hormone and testosterone, though, their use in professional cycling is legal – well, in training and recovery anyway. Although there are strict guidelines. The UCI (cycling's international governing body) don't permit socks above mid-calf height in racing. Any higher and you'll be contravening UCI rules; in essence, you're a sock doper. Any length goes, though, when the stage is finished.

It's hard to pinpoint the exact Eureka moment when compression socks gravitated from the hospital to sport but the consensus suggests it's down to a 1987 study in the *American Journal Of Physical Medicine*, when doctors Michael Berry and Robert McMurray revealed that athletes wearing compression stockings recovered faster than athletes not wearing them.

'Compression wear has a multitude of benefits,' says Akbar de Medici, medical director at Compression Advisory who have worked with a number of elite sporting teams. 'They include improving venous return to speed up recovery and reduce muscle damage.'

That muscle damage is less applicable to cyclists because that's more down to restricting muscle oscillation (the vibration of muscles due to repetitive impact), which is more applicable to the weight-bearing sport of running. Venous return (speeding up blood flow back to the heart) is important, though, and something to remember when mocking Contador and co. wandering around the paddock in their high-school socks.

A by-product of riding is free radicals. These are atoms or groups of atoms with an odd number of electrons, making them unstable. In search of electron parity, they attack different parts of the body, including DNA, skin, hair and muscle tissue. Each day, free radical attack happens on a huge scale. Add in the extra metabolic cost and breathing rate of competing at the Tour and there's an internal war going on in riders' bodies that will impede subsequent performance if they don't whip out their defences. By wearing compression socks and warming down slowly, the riders begin the process of flushing out these toxins and flooding oxygenated blood around the body.

Compression socks purport to work because your body has what could be termed a 'second heart'. This is a system of muscles, veins and valves in the calf and foot that work together to send deoxygenated, toxic blood back up to the heart and lungs for cleansing and oxygenation. Compression wear simply gives it a helping hand.

'But it has to feature graduated pressure or they won't work,' says Mike Martin of compression-wear company 2XU. 'If, for example, there's greater pressure at the calves than ankle, they won't provide improved venous return and so won't improve recovery.' That's why fit is so important. Compression is measured in millimetres of mercury (mmHg), which is a unit of pressure and more commonly applied to blood pressure. A normal resting blood pressure is 120/80mmHg. The top figure (systolic) is pressure of blood away from the heart; the bottom figure (diastolic) is pressure of blood back to the heart.

'That blood pressure obviously lowers away from the heart and is why many compression manufacturers settle on around 22mmHg at the ankle and 18mmHg at the thigh, but these values vary between manufacturers,' reads a BASES (British Association of Sport and Exercise Sciences) official statement on compression. Sizing is vital and is why bespoke socks designed to the rider's calf dimensions are common, though not essential.

'The problem is, commercial models often don't apply compression high enough to elicit the physiological effect you're after,' says BMC Racing sports

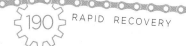

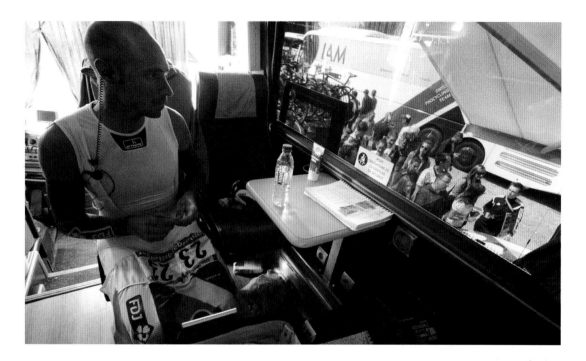

## CHAPTER 10

△ Team buses are a place to recover and discuss stage tactics

scientist David Bailey. 'That's why predominantly we use customised garments. Originally the riders were simply measured around the circumference of the leg at different points, but now they're scanned with a laser scanner and knitted to fit.'

'I've had custom made and out-of-the box versions from several brands and I wouldn't say one was more effective than the other,' retorts Bookwalter. 'For me, they both worked.'

Once the riders have concluded their stage duties, which can include media commitments and urine tests at doping control, it's time to step onto their respective team buses for not only transporting to their next Ibis, but also to continue the recovery process.

## THE TEAM KITCHEN

Mind you, we're not talking a run-down white van here – team buses are now state-of-the-art performance vehicles. Again, Team Sky elevated things to a higher level when they rolled into town with their Death Star, which reportedly took 9,000 man hours and four months to kit out. As well as a cinema screen (to replay the stage), there are personalised seats that electronically shift back, which again is good for recovery and flushing out toxins. There's also a kitchen, fridge, showers, hand gel sanitisers, massage tables and meeting room. There's even mood lighting to enhance the rider's focus.

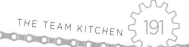

Team Sky also rolled out a new kitchen truck at the 2015 Giro d'Italia, which they drove over to the Tour de France. It featured two ovens, a range of blenders – some Sky branded though not yet for sale – a rice cooker and a dining area where Froome and crew ate. It's impressive; though, for once, dwarfed by another team's – Bora-Argon 18's kitchen truck. It measures 19 metres in length and includes a glass cube and trailer for the world to observe the alchemy within. It's a different world for Kim Rokkjaer, who's head chef of Trek-Segafredo and has to make do with sharing a hotel kitchen with the head chef of whichever hotel Cancellara and team are staying in.

'Do I have kitchen envy?' he says. 'Not a bit of it. It'd drive me mad working in a truck all day.' Instead, Rokkjaer liaises with the respective hotel manager and hotel chef beforehand to ensure there'll be a section of the kitchen reserved for him.

Team Dimension Data also don't have a separate kitchen truck. Instead, their team bus doubles as a kitchen, featuring two hob rings and a tiny sink. It's still large enough for their performance biochemist Rob Child to accelerate rider recovery through post-stage nutrition. 'My approach to nutrition is unique and based on targeting specific chemical pathways and then identifying foods and nutrients that are capable of delivering the desired metabolic effects,' he says. 'It's very different to the approach of real chefs, who focus on palatability and presentation and have nutritionists tell them the ideal nutrient composition, but not biochemistry or physiological effects. For me, the difficult part is incorporating the required nutrients into a package that is palatable and convenient enough that it can be delivered under race conditions.'

'What can happen with the riders is that they eat healthy snacks on the bus and a really big meal in the evening, which is one strategy,' Child continues. 'But I try to get the guys to have a meal on the bus, too, though it depends on how far the transfer is to the hotel from the race finish.

'Look at some stages of the Tour,' he adds. 'Often stages finish at 5–5.30pm. If it's a mountain stage, some of the guys will come in 45 minutes later than the first riders. So maybe leave at 6.30pm and a two-hour transfer. Hotel at 8.30pm, followed by massage, so it might be 9.30–10pm when they eat which is over four hours after finishing the stage. That's not great for recovery.'

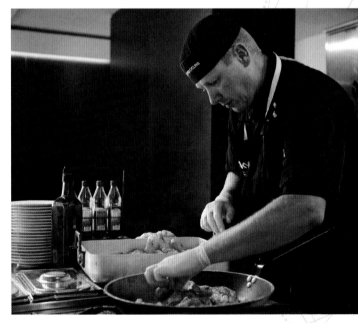

▽ Team Sky chef Soren Kristiansen prepares food for the team

So on-board the team bus he cooks simple food high in carbohydrate, protein and antioxidants. 'So there would be fresh fruit salad, homemade rice pudding, pasta with pesto and pine nuts, chicken, garlic and tuna.'

In fact, conjuring up the most nutritionally dense and tastiest 'fuel' has become a challenge amongst the teams with Tinkoff Sport's Hannah Grant and Team Sky's Soren Kristiansen, both chefs, delivering a Twitter food-off on a near daily basis. From Grant you might have chicken tagine with shallot and zucchini on a bed of rice. Kristiansen will retaliate with guacamole basil pesto alongside a fennel and cucumber salad with baked beets. It serves to fuel the riders and whet the appetites of their thousands of followers but, logistically, it looks a nightmare.

'Our kitchen truck is big so we can stock up on a lot of ingredients before we arrive in France,' says Grant. 'As for the fresh produce, I tend to source locally. Usually I contact the hotels to tell them I'm coming. Nicer hotels have nice produce so I ask if I can have some of that, or if they could recommend a nice fishmonger or nice butcher so we can trace it back to avoid contamination and then choose from them.'

The process of cooking is also a factor in accelerating recovery. 'We really only grill and steam,' says BMC Racing's nutritionist Judith Haudum. 'Frying food simply adds fat and that takes longer for the riders to process. So during the Tour we're more about good-quality carbs and protein.'

Buses also feature a shower for the riders to cool down and clean up. A few teams might also have ice baths but the jury is out on whether these should be used for anything more than cooling core temperature during a hot stage (see Chapter 11).

'I'm not a big fan of anything that's anti-inflammatory, which would include ice baths,' explains David Bailey, sports scientist at BMC Racing, who has had a paper on the subject featured in the *Journal of Sports Science*. 'What I've discovered is that they may have a temporary, acute beneficial effect but, in the long term, may be harming the adaptation process. I've seen a benefit in perceived soreness for two or three days afterwards, but ultimately, I feel it can blunt adaptation.'

The idea that a recovery ice bath might not be such a good idea is down to icing suppressing the cell-signalling response that regulates muscle growth. It's an area exercise physiologist Jonathan Peake and his colleagues at Queensland University of Technology in Brisbane, Australia, examined in 2014. They put two groups of men on a biweekly resistance-training plan. The first group took ice baths – around 10 minutes in water at 50°F – after each session; the second group did a low-intensity cool-down on a bicycle like Team Sky. The results showed that the ice group didn't improve their strength results to the level of the non-ice group.

Then again, another 2014 study, this time by Shona Halson of the Australian Institute of Sport, found that ice baths weren't detrimental to adaptation and improved aspects of cycling performance, like mean and sprint power output.

Once on the bus, many riders, including Chris Froome, might also use Normatec's compression system. (In the past, Froome has tweeted a photo of him

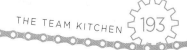

recovering in the Normatec device.) This is a tight-like-system that sends waves of pressure from the ankles up to the thigh, like compression socks the aim being to push out toxins. 'I try and use one every day at a Grand Tour,' says Bookwalter.

A more proven recovery technique adopted by all is the daily massage. These can last up to an hour and continue the process of flushing out toxins, as well as stretching out leg muscles that have been shortening throughout the day. The importance of massage to a Tour rider's recovery plan is revealed in the 'Massage to Paris' box on the next page.

How all of these technologies are integrated is very much a team-specific approach. But, according to sports scientist at the Australian Institute of Sport and Orica GreenEdge David Martin, key is giving the rider responsibility for their decisions and actions. 'The Tour de France is a big game of abuse but we feel it's better if the athlete can choose the kind of technology they want to use to temper that abuse. So instead of saying, "use these compression socks, they'll make you recover better", we say after the race, "you can use medical-grade compression hosiery or you can use the 2XU compression, which you can use longer. Or you can mix and match." By them taking the lead, we can work with them a lot easier. Making choices is very powerful. If you choose something yourself, you'll believe in it more. And never underestimate the power of belief.'

# SLEEP YOUR WAY TO VICTORY

One recovery technique every rider, every team, every scientist believes in is sleep. It's often said that the rider who wins the Tour is the one who's slept the best. Which perhaps makes it surprising that sleep is one of the most under-researched areas in professional cycling, especially when you consider the mental and physical regeneration that occurs during the night. Sleep improves glucose metabolism, cognitive performance, regulates appetite and, perhaps the most important when riding with eight other riders each day, it improves mood.

'But one of the most important benefits of sleep is it releases growth hormone,' says Shona Halson, head of recovery at the Australian Institute of Sport who's worked with Orica GreenEdge. 'That helps aspects like muscle repair, which is clearly important over 21 stages.'

Historically, cycling's association with nocturnal activities is confined to the questionable moral antics of five-time Tour winner Jacques Anquetil – who enjoyed a *ménage à trois* with his wife and step-daughter before having an affair with his step-son's wife – and doping. During the bad old days blood transfusions or injected EPO thickened the blood to such an extent that during a period of rest, like overnight, the lack of circulation could lower blood pressure so much that you might never wake up. That's why it was common to find professionals awakening in the night for a quick set of squats or a turbo session to get their blood pumping again.

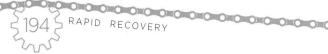

# Massage to Paris

○ Professional riders have relied on the firm hands, elbows and even knees of their team's soigneurs for years. Every rider at the Tour de France follows a similar routine: race, transfer to hotel, massage, eat and bed. It's like clockwork.

'At our team, we split the nine riders between four soigneurs,' says Trek-Segafredo soigneur Sabine Lueber, who worked for the team at the 2015 edition. 'Each rider has one hour of massage, and they swear by it.'

Sports massage purports to achieve a plethora of multi-stage benefits, including: dilating blood vessels to accelerate the removal of waste products and enhance the speed of oxygen delivery to the muscles; relieving muscle tension and soreness; and improving the muscle's range of motion – key when pedalling for over 200km the following day.

Research conducted by scientists from the Buck Institute for Research on Aging at McMaster University in Ontario, Canada, also showed that massage reduces inflammation of muscles and promotes the growth of new mitochondria, the energy-producing units in cells.

'Daily massage really helps the riders but it's very painful. If it's not, it's not working,' adds Lueber, before explaining that applied pressure is rider-specific. 'Someone like Frank [Schleck], he's a climber so has very skinny legs so you don't have to press too hard. Someone like Fabian [Cancellara], though, who's more of a sprinter and classics rider, he has really big thighs so it's harder to dig into the muscle. That's why I have to apply a lot of pressure.'

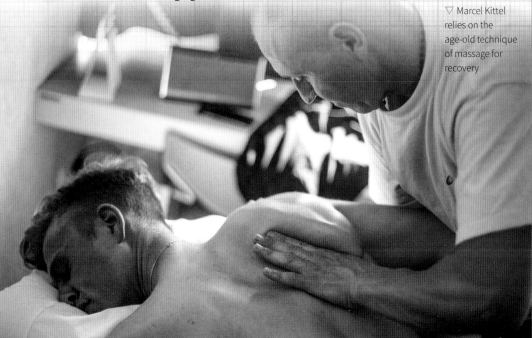

▽ Marcel Kittel relies on the age-old technique of massage for recovery

It seems, though, that teams are catching on to the importance of sleep, especially during the demands of a Grand Tour. At the 2015 Giro d'Italia, Sky's race leader, Ritchie Porte, slept in a motorhome outside the team's hotel every night so that 'the Australian wasn't stressed by different rooms and unfamiliarity'.

'We got the idea from Moto GP drivers,' a Sky spokesperson said at the Giro. 'The benefit is the familiarity. We studied the impact of different hotels every day for three weeks of a Grand Tour and it showed to be stressful. This lessens the stress.'

Sadly, Porte didn't make it to Milan, withdrawing after time penalties and a crash put him out of contention. The UCI weren't impressed, either, immediately amending 'article 2.2.010' to read 'riders must stay in the hotels provided by the organiser throughout the entire duration of the race'.

Riders' accommodation hit the headlines once more at the 2015 Tour de France. On the second rest day in Gap, Oleg Tinkov and Alberto Contador complained to the world's media about the lack of air conditioning and high temperatures in their Best Western hotel. 'This is not the conditions the riders deserve,' Tinkov told a sweltering pack of journalists including myself. 'It's not acceptable for such a big event. They race under the sun for six hours and they come back to this.' Tour organisers ASO say they visit every hotel the teams will use, rate them on a scale of one to five, and then randomly distribute the hotels so that everyone gets a share of the good, poor and downright boiling.

Sky has form in the area of sleep, making the news for bringing their own mattresses, duvets and pillows to races. Apparently it takes each soigneur an hour to pack up each of the rider's bedtime tools … before offloading at the next hotel.

'Sky is probably at the extreme end – a mattress topper would suffice – but if you have the money and people, then why not?' says Shona Halson at the AIS, who has studied sleep for over 10 years and knows its importance for Tour riders. 'What we do know is that during the different phases of sleep, there are different focuses on recovery. The first half of the night there's a tendency for the body to prioritise physical recovery; the second half moves to brain recovery. Although both happen throughout the night, there's a definite shift in priority. We believe the slow-wave sleep, which is stages three and four (deep sleep), that's where most of the physical repair happens.'

> A meticulous sleep strategy should become an ever-more important area of research and application for riders at the Tour.
>
> **Sophie KILLER,** *physiologist*

How much sleep a rider needs – and actually gets – is a highly individual thing. A look at other sports shows the potential discrepancy between athletes. Roger Federer reportedly can't swing a racquet unless he's had 12 hours; Usain Bolt sleeps 8–10 hours each night according to Zeo, a now-defunct company that sold sleep-monitoring devices. What is clear is that the demands of a three-week stage race can take their toll.

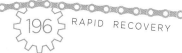

'Many riders can start to struggle with sleep as the Tour progress, especially during the third and final week where they're severely fatigued and they hit the Alps', says Halson. 'We'd certainly ensure they were activating the correct recovery techniques, like nutrition and massage, although some might look to sleeping medication if they're really struggling.'

'One or two bad nights isn't such an issue,' Halson continues. 'Four or five and we do begin to see potential effects on performance. You'd observe decreases in power output, reaction time and decision-making, which obviously isn't ideal if you're shoulder to shoulder with many other riders. Of course, you can use caffeine, legal stimulants like energy drinks to try and keep you awake, and keep performance up, which might be okay if you only have three days to go. It's when Paris is a long way off and you feel that you have no control, that's when riders find it difficult.'

Research undertaken in 2015 by physiologists Asker Jeukendrup and Sophie Killer in the United Kingdom examined the impact of high-intensity exercise and carbohydrate intake on the sleep patterns of cyclists over a simulated multi-stage race. They took well-trained cyclists with $VO_2$ maxes around 72–73 and put them through two blocks of nine-day intensive training. Each involved four to five hours of indoor and outdoor interval sets. ('It was hard – we made grown men cry,' says Killer.) In fact, the only thing that varied was the composition of training nutrition.

'We wanted to see if feeding with a high-carbohydrate strategy during training altered sleep compared to moderate-carbohydrate intake,' explains Killer. The results showed that carbohydrate intake didn't produce significant results. What was significant, however, was that not surprisingly the cyclists spent longer in bed – from an average of 456 minutes per night to 509 minutes – after the block of high-intensity training. Kitted out with sleep monitors, the researchers also measured the quality of the riders' sleep and observed that, though time in bed was up, the quality of sleep dropped, as did their mood. 'As the study progressed, this had an impact on the quality of their performance, namely it went down,' says Killer.

Killer concluded that a meticulous sleep strategy should become an ever-more important area of research and application for riders at the Tour. At the English Institute of Sport, many of the track-and-field athletes Killer works with nap for 20 minutes on race day, swallowing a caffeine pill just before they get their head down so that when they wake up, they're buzzing and in a heightened state of preparation.

Naps have been used by such esteemed figures as Albert Einstein and Napoleon, and have been shown to restore alertness, enhance performance and reduce mistakes. A study at NASA on military pilots and astronauts found that a 40-minute nap improved performance by 34 per cent and alertness by 100 per cent.

'Clearly a nap isn't overly useful for Tour riders before a stage because they usually start in the morning or at lunchtime,' adds Killer. 'However, it's something Grand Tour riders can play around with. If a stage finishes around 4–5pm, they could experiment with a quick nap during the transfer to the hotel as, after massage and

 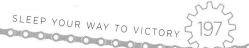

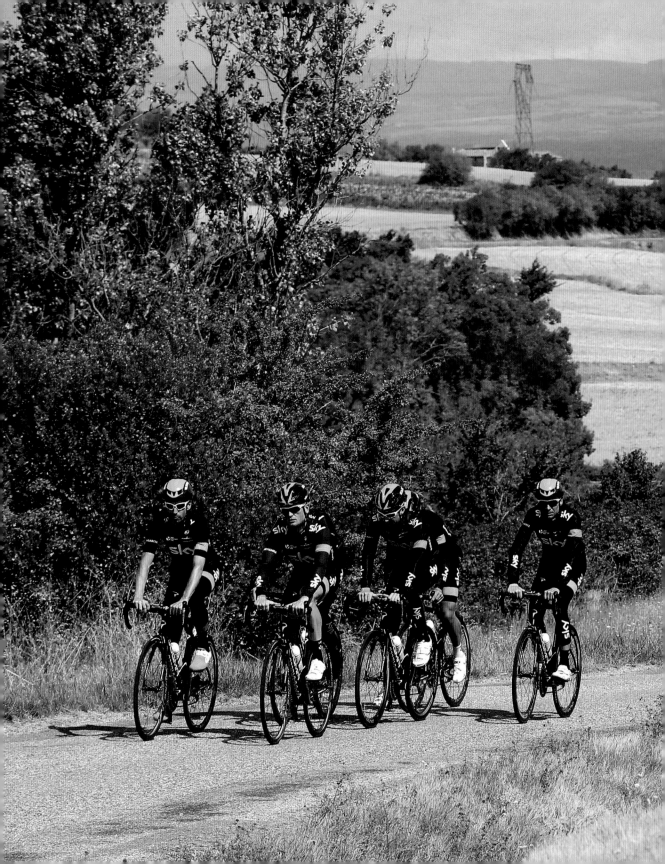

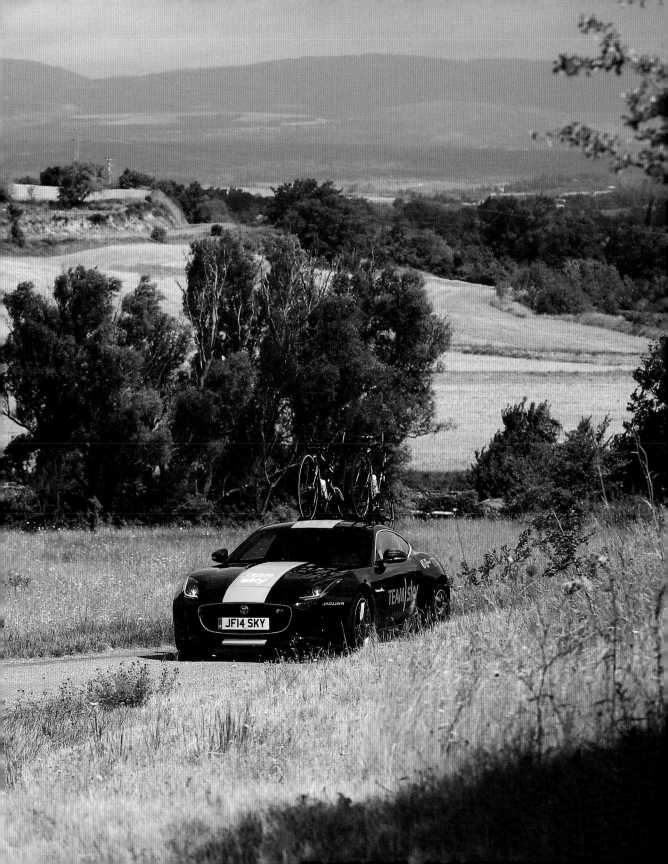

eating, they probably won't sleep until around 11pm. This is where areas such as brain entrainment come in. We use headphones that produce these sonar pulses. The idea is that it channels different parts of the brain that are involved in relaxation but might also simply work as a distraction.'

Brain entrainment's also an area that Halson has looked into, though she focuses on proven strategies for now. 'There are many interventions that can help a rider sleep, including eye masks and ear plugs, the right temperature of the room, reducing noise and light. Staying off bright-light devices like smartphones and iPads is useful, too. That light stimulates the body clock and tells you to stay awake. You want as dark a room as possible in the hour before bed because it primes the body for sleep.'

Nutrition plays an important role in sleep quality, too. Milk continues to be a bedtime favourite for many riders and teams thanks not only to muscle-repairing protein but also down to the amino acid tryptophan, which helps you to sleep. And then, of course, there are the two rest days where the riders can sit back, doff a cocktail and top up their tan … Not a bit of it.

## IMPORTANCE OF THE REST DAY

'Rest days can be very hard to manage,' says BMC Racing sports scientist David Bailey. 'Riders are the opposite of guys who do no exercise in that they've been exercising so intensely that when they stop, it's actually physically and psychologically hard for them.'

After stage 16 of the 2012 Vuelta, Katusha's Joaquim Rodríguez led Alberto Contador by 28 seconds. Rodríguez had led the race for 13 stages, frequently fending off Contador's repeated attacks. The next day was a rest day before the riders returned for stage 17 – 187.3km between Santander and Fuente Dé. Unlike several of the previous days, stage 17 was viewed as relatively safe for Rodríguez with only the occasional mountain punctuating a predominantly flat route. That didn't matter to Contador who broke Rodriguez on the flat before pulling further away on the category-two ascent to Fuente Dé. Rodriguez looked sluggish after the rest day losing 2 minutes 38 seconds to his Spanish rival and with it the chance of his first Grand Tour title.

'Part of the problem when you have a recovery day is that the body is over-recovering,' says Bailey. 'The body's become used to turning over a huge number of calories and carbohydrate every day, so when the rider is inactive, if they don't temper their calorie intake, you see what's called a supercompensation of calorie stores.'

What is supercompensation? Well, every gram of carbohydrate stored in the body brings with it three grams of water. If riders eat the same amount of carbohydrate on a rest day, without expending all that energy, they're left with an excess.

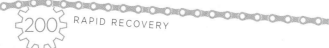

This makes the cells swell up and, when they do, metabolic processes become inefficient and the riders put on weight.

'I remember when I was at British Cycling, we saw it worst when you took a road cyclist to the track,' says Bailey. 'I remember one year Geraint Thomas went from 74kg to 80kg before the world championships and that was all fluid. In one week! The problem would be similar to taking a marathon runner and getting him to run a middle-distance race. Geraint changed from riding four or five hours a day to just an hour top-end work. It left his cells and weight swelling right up, which wasn't a huge problem on the track but is an issue on the road and, in particular, on the mountain stages.'

Bailey has discovered that Normatec, which increases blood pressure from the ankles through to the calves and thighs, is a useful tool for alleviating this situation because it keeps the blood flowing at a high volume and doesn't let the inactive cells swell with water. Calorie reduction also helps, of course, with riders consuming less than normal during the rest day, refuelling in the evening like they would during the stages in preparation for the following day's exertions. Every rider also heads out for a low-intensity 60–90-minute ride to try and reduce the issues of supercompensation. Bailey also suggests that at the 2014 Tour, one team tried to induce dehydration in their riders on the rest day in an effort to reduce added weight from water content. 'The problem with that is you're not sure how much water is in the blood plasma compared to the cells so it's potentially a risky strategy,' he says. In other words, while dehydration might reduce the water content of the cells and so not add excess weight or sluggishness to the rider, lowering the water content in the blood plasma can lead to inefficient metabolic processes and a slowing of recovery.

Away from the Tour, apps are having an impact on how riders manage fatigue levels. 'I've experimented with a recovery programme called Restwise,' says Bookwalter. 'It gives you a recovery score on how you're feeling.'

The theory behind Restwise follows this logical process: they identify the research-based markers that relate to recovery and overtraining, determine their importance, create an algorithm that collects the data and puts it through a meaningful calculation and then generates a score that tells the rider how prepared the body is for training. If it's well-prepared, you can work hard; ill-prepared, either have the day off or keep the intensity low. For more on Restwise, see the '21st-century recovery' box, page 205.

'Heart rate also has its place in recovery,' adds Bookwalter. 'It's easily measured on and off the bike, when you wake up and at numerous points throughout the day. If your heart rate is significantly up on normal, that's often a sign your body's struggling and you're not recovering sufficiently.'

But one of the most common tools used by professional teams to manage fatigue takes us back to TrainingPeaks – the company we first met in Chapter 1. 'On our system, I'd say a recovery day is as important as the hardest workout,' says

 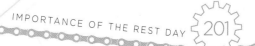

co-founder Dirk Friel. 'When you have fitness level and subtract fatigue, that's form. The worst thing possible is for a rider to show up to the Tour and fatigue is higher than fitness. We call that a "negative training balance". The problem is that fatigue grows three to four times faster than fitness.'

TrainingPeaks use what they call a 'training stress score' based on the quality of bike session, which is down to factors like intensity, duration and frequency of workouts. That information's then put into the performance management chart, which can measure training load and training stress balance. It then gives you a score based on all these variables that'll tell the rider if they're recovered or not.

'It's something that's benefited my performance,' says Tinkoff Sport's Michael Rogers, who has nine Grand Tour's worth of TrainingPeaks data stored away. 'Mind you, it doesn't help afterwards as it always takes me a month to recover from the Tour de France. It doesn't help that the weekend after the Tour I'll usually race down in the Basque country doing San Sebastián. I've done that race nine or ten times as we're committed to racing it but I'm often physically going through the motions. Your legs just turn on memory. But that's individual. Some guys thrive on a broad base of work and can recover after a week.'

Rogers also credits the fact professionals race less than they used to for managing fatigue. 'Most do about 80 days a year now, which is a lot less than just five years ago when the majority of riders were completing well over 100 race days a year. The problem is, when you race so much it's really hard to measure intensity and fatigue.'

For how effective fewer race days can be Rogers gives the example of Bradley Wiggins's Tour de France win in 2012. Wiggins was only racing every three weeks. 'It's about the training, too,' he adds. 'I remember at HTC where we could ride for six hours, and ride well for four hours but be dead for two. That'd just make you more fatigued for the day after. A lot of pro cyclists seemed to create self-esteem and self-confidence based on hours rather than quality. Thankfully, the sport has learnt that quality eclipses quantity.'

Fatigue management has become the buzzword among sports scientists at professional cycling teams, and is perhaps the strongest sign that the EPO era of Armstrong and Riis is, if not totally behind cycling, certainly far less prevalent than in the 2000s. A chemical shopping list including EPO and steroids would forge superhuman competitors who recorded superhuman times. As it transpired, they were far from superhuman. Now, with the majority of riders seemingly working with the physiology that Mother Nature gave them, managing fatigue has become a vital area for performance improvements.

In an interview UCI president Brian Cookson gave to Agence France-Presse after the 2015 Tour, the Englishman said that levels of fatigue felt by the riders was proof that anti-doping measures like the blood passport are having the desired effect. 'I think we saw that riders during the Tour de France were very tired and one

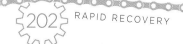

of the causes, in my opinion, is the increased efficiency of doping controls,' Cookson explained, presumably alluding to the time gains Quintana made into Froome as the race approached Paris. It's a notion backed up by just one positive test from the race after Katusha's Luca Paolini tested positive for cocaine in the opening week.

Managing a rider's fatigue levels is vital to success. Though riders don't race as much as their cycling ancestors, who've been reported to have competed for 250 days a year, as Trek-Segafredo's Tim Vanderjeugd told me at the 2015 Tour, 'They still race for 12,000–14,000km and train for 15,000–20,000km each year.' An annual tally of 34,000km of cycling is reason enough to play around with scientifically based equipment, training and nutrition regimes.

## 21st-century recovery

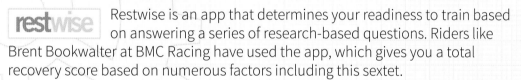 Restwise is an app that determines your readiness to train based on answering a series of research-based questions. Riders like Brent Bookwalter at BMC Racing have used the app, which gives you a total recovery score based on numerous factors including this sextet.

● **Resting heart rate:** Daily variations of resting heart rate of around 5 per cent are common and not usually associated with fatigue or stress. However, increases of greater than 5 per cent are reported in athletes who are severely fatigued.

● **Body mass:** Rapid loss of weight compromises the body's ability to repair itself after intense training. A body mass loss of 2 per cent or more can adversely affect cognitive and physical performance.

● **Sleep:** Although every rider's sleep requirements differ, many sleep specialists gravitate around the 8-hour mark as the healthy average. When a rider regularly sleeps less than this, recovery will be negatively influenced. Either, or both, sleep volume and quantity can be affected, which can undermine adaptation.

● **Appetite:** Riders' appetites decrease with fatigue, which can result in a negative energy balance. Inadequate carbohydrate intake can lead to impaired performance and potential illness through a depleted immune system.

● **Muscle soreness:** Delayed onset of muscle soreness (DOMS) is thought to be a result of microscopic tearing of the muscle fibres, resulting in intra-muscular inflammation. DOMS is a natural reaction to high-intensity training. On the other hand, persistent muscle soreness may indicate an increased risk of overtraining.

● **Previous day's performance:** Ultimately, this is the most valid indicator of fatigue. While brief periods of underperformance are expected in a training programme or three-week stage race, prolonged underperformance is a reliable indicator of severe fatigue or overtraining.

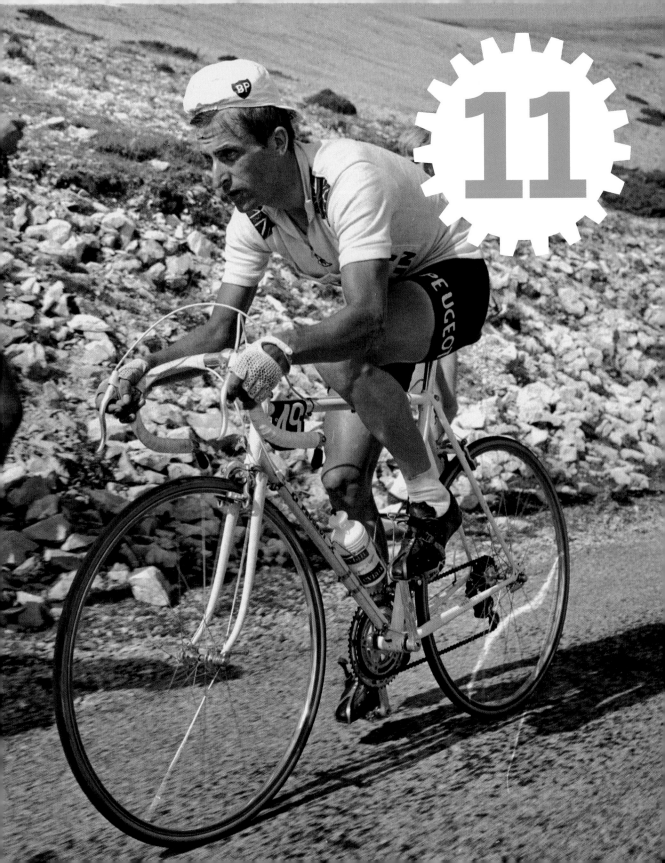

# BEAT THE HEAT

'It was an incredibly hot day with temperatures in excess of 35°C. I thought my head was going to explode when I arrived at the base of the final climb.' The words of Team Sky's Geraint Thomas after Richie Porte – who'd replaced Chris Froome as leader following the Brit's withdrawal at the end of stage five – and his team had struggled on stage 13's mountainous route to Chamrousse, effectively ending their hopes of winning the 2014 Tour de France. 'I'd been drinking three bottles [of water and carbohydrate drink] every hour – around 1.5 litres – to keep myself hydrated and ride at threshold,' Thomas continued.

Stifling heat also suffocated many stages of the 2015 Tour. When the riders reached the Pyrenees, temperatures soared to nearly 40°C. Both Vincenzo Nibali and Alberto Contador complained of being 'unable to breathe on the climbs'. On the 13th stage from Muret to Rodez, roadside temperature measured 61°C – the record stands at 63°C set in 2010. FDJ's Thibaut Pinot, who finished third in 2014, suffered so badly on the 188km 11th stage from Pau to Vallée de Saint-Savin that he finished over 21 minutes behind stage winner Rafał Majka. 'I've come to realise these last few days that as soon as it gets hot, I quickly lose energy,' said the 25-year-old. 'The heat is a mountain.'

It's one thing riding in the heat – it's another riding at maximum effort in the Tour de France while climbing over 3,000m in a stage after numerous days of racing beforehand. Some days can be comparable to riding in a sauna, leading to over-heating, hyperthermia or even worse.

Britain's Tom Simpson entered the 1967 edition in good form after winning two stages of the Vuelta – which used to take place in April – and GC at Paris–Nice. In search of securing his financial future (winning a stage in those days guaranteed the winner entry into lucrative post-Tour criteriums), he harboured ambitions of a top-three finish or wearing *le maillot jaune* for at least one day. He'd targeted three stages to attack including the 13th over the monumental Mont Ventoux, whose backdrop offers little vegetation to provide shade from the heat.

◁ Tom Simpson tragically died ascending Mont-Ventoux climb in 1967. Reportedly, road temperature reached 54°C

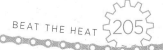

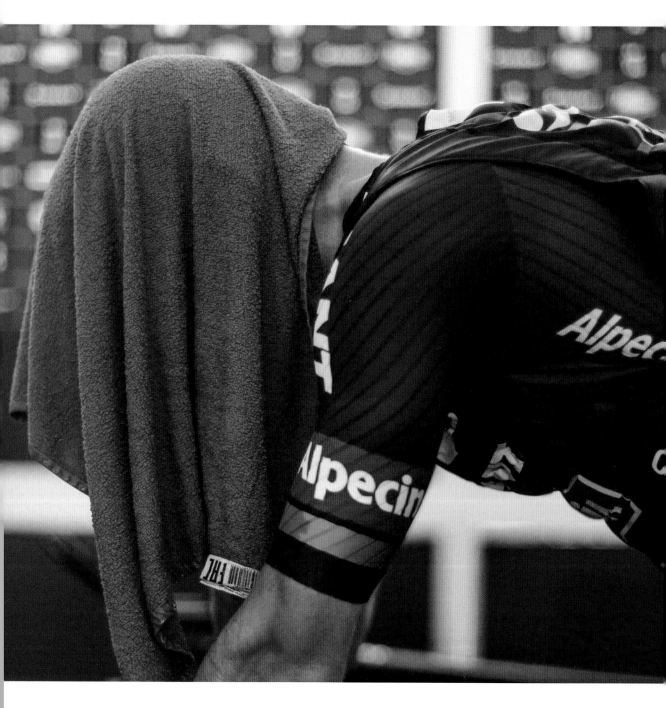

△ Giant-Alpecin emlpoy cold towels and
ice vests when preparing for time trials

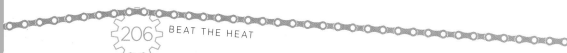

As dawn broke on stage 13, Tour doctor Pierre Dumas noted the imminent hot day ahead and reportedly told journalist Pierre Chany, 'If the boys stick their nose in a "topette" [bag of drugs] today, we could have a death on our hands.' As the riders lined up in Marseille for the 211.5km stage, a fellow journalist noticed Simpson's tired state – he'd been struck with diarrhoea and stomach pains just days before – and asked if the heat was a problem. 'It's not the heat,' came Simpson's reply. 'It's the Tour.'

Temperature reports from the race aren't accurate but some accounts suggest it reached a near unbelievable 54°C. At Bédoin, where the Ventoux climb begins, Simpson is said to have stopped off at a local café to fill up on whiskey and pastis. That seems foolhardy now but, at the time, Tour regulations permitted the riders' support staff to give the riders liquid only at certain intervals; there was also a belief among the peloton that alcohol taken during the race did you no harm because it was quickly sweated out. The legendary 580km Bordeaux–Paris race, completed in one stretch, saw many teams prescribe the following drinks plan: port, white wine, eau-de-vie (fruit brandy) and champagne.

Simpson settled into the leading group as the riders began the ascent of Ventoux but soon slipped back to a group of chasers. He then began to lose control of his bike, zigzagging all over the road before collapsing. With help from his team manager, he remounted but collapsed again 500 metres later. He was pronounced dead at 5.40pm that same day. England's *Daily Mail* reported, 'He died in the saddle, slowly asphyxiated by intense effort in a heatwave after taking methylamphetamine drugs and alcohol.'

# EVOLUTION OF HYDRATION

Hydration strategies evolved, as did the use of illegal performance enhancers, moving from stimulants (amphetamines were only declared illegal in the mid-1960s) to drugs designed to fortify, notably growth hormone and EPO (erythropoietin). Gone are the days when teams would see water as extra weight: 'The goal now is that riders don't finish the stage in a dehydrated state and that means staying within 2 per cent of their starting body weight,' explains Judith Haudum, nutritionist at BMC Racing. 'If we fail to achieve that aim, their performance will be impaired.'

So for a rider like America's Tejay van Garderen, whose racing weight hovers around 70kg, that'd mean losing 1.4kg. Any more, the theory goes, will result in a catalogue of negative side effects: an increase in core temperature, reduced muscle contraction, insufficient carbohydrate absorption and poor decision-making through mental fatigue.

'Sweat and electrolyte losses are huge in a three-week stage race like the Tour. With all that going on you need to maintain blood volume,' adds sports scientist

 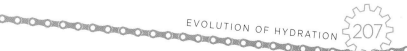

# Electrolytes masterclass

O Andy Blow is the founder of H2Pro Hydrate, a company who test a rider's sweat rate and then determine how much sodium they should ingest when exercising. In the past they've worked with Garmin-Sharp. Here he charts the key electrolytes involved in a Tour rider maintaining peak performance. The table charts values for each electrolyte and how the heat impacts upon respective levels.

● **Sodium:** Sodium (Na+) is the most abundant and possibly the most important electrolyte in the body. This positively charged electrolyte is primarily found outside the cell and is key to muscle contraction and nerve conduction. It's also essential for the transport of water within the body; your body can't excrete and move water without sodium. Blood sodium loss and gains are regulated by the kidney, with messages sent from the brain to increase salt intake or drink more water. Normal blood levels are maintained between 135–145mmol per litre.

● **Potassium:** Potassium (K+) is a positively charged electrolyte found inside of cells. It regulates the electrical integrity of the cell membrane so is important in nerve conduction. It also helps to transport glucose into the cell so is crucial for energy generation. Blood levels of potassium are regulated between 4.5–5.5mmol per litre. Low blood potassium (hypokalaemia) is usually due to diarrhoea, fasting and taking diuretics.

● **Magnesium:** Magnesium (Mg+) is necessary in every cell for enzyme reaction, as well as muscle contraction and energy production. Prolonged exercise and training with poor diet can lead to depletion, which could lead to dizziness, fatigue and depression.

● **Calcium:** Calcium is (Ca++) involved in muscle contraction and relaxation, nerve contraction, hormonal secretion and blood clotting. Your body stores vast supplies in bones, which are tapped into when needed. A good diet, including dairy products (normally fortified with Vitamin D to help calcium absorption), will supply enough calcium for health and well-being.

## H2ProHydrate table

| ELECTROLYTE | TYPICAL DAILY INTAKE (mg) | TYPICAL ABSORPTION EFFICIENCY | TYPICAL SWEAT LOSSES PER LITRE (mg) | LOSS IN LITRES OF SWEAT TO BE DEFICIENT | DEFICIENCY POSSIBLE BY SWEATING? |
|---|---|---|---|---|---|
| Sodium* | 4,000 | >90% | 230-1,700 | 4 | Yes |
| Potassium | 2,700 | >90% | 150 | 16 | No |
| Calcium | 500 | 30% | 28 | 5 | Possible |
| Magnesium | 300 | 10-70% | 8.3-14.2 | 15 | No |

*Sweating 2 l/hr in a not race would mean that in as little as 2 hours you would deplete your daily intake of sodium. Considering that there are no useable reserves of sodium in the body this would need to be replaced as you exercise.
Source: *Nutrition for Sports* 2nd edition, Dr Arnie Baker

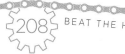

Andy Blow, an expert on the role sodium plays in the body during cycling (see the 'Electrolytes masterclass' box for more information). A typical adult has a blood volume of around five litres, but that figure's partly dictated by the amount of water consumed. At the Tour, riders can easily sweat a litre each hour and that needs to be replaced. If not, blood volume will drop below five litres, making the blood more viscous and harder to pump around the body.

This reduced blood volume lowers the rider's cardiac output (amount of blood pumped by the heart each minute). So if a rider's heart pumps out 100 millilitres (ml) of blood each beat and their heart rate is 100bpm, their cardiac output is 10,000ml each minute. When dehydrated, blood volume can drop markedly, so despite an increase in heart rate, cardiac output falls. For instance, dehydration might see a rider's heart rate rise to 130bpm but the heart might only pump out 40ml per beat, so the cardiac output is 5,200ml per minute. As blood supplies oxygen to working muscles, clearly this is detrimental to performance.

Out on the roads, the performance repercussions are highlighted by a 2007 study from Dr Dan Judelson of California State University who showed that

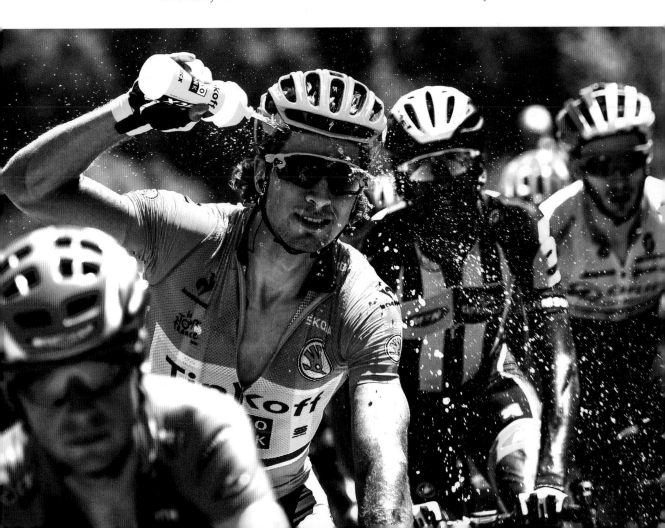

a sustained state of dehydration impaired strength, power and high-intensity muscular endurance by 2 per cent, 3 per cent and 10 per cent, respectively. Those are significant figures, especially that 10 per cent drop in muscular endurance. Muscular endurance is vital for sustained efforts, like a breakaway. Lose 10 per cent and the Tour rider could well be swept up by the broom wagon (the vehicle that follows the race to pick up stragglers who are unable to make the cut-off time).

What kind of temperatures are the riders facing during a hot French summer day? Often the commentators refer to a particular temperature, but that can often be far removed from the heat experienced by the riders out on the road. Commentators refer to 'shade temperature' measured by something called a 'Stevenson screen'. This is a meteorological instrument housed within a shelter so doesn't capture the full intensity of what's being radiated to the peloton. Black strips of tarmac absorb the heat from the sun easily and by the time the day's stage starts, road surface can easily reach 50–80°C. In turn, the air directly above is heated up like a kettle, so when the temperature in the shade is 32–40°C, that could equate to 50°C or more for the cyclist.

Sometimes, the Tour roads reach such extreme temperatures that the tarmac can become sticky, catching out unsuspecting riders as they descend at 50mph-plus. In 2003, ONCE's Joseba Beloki was in second place overall and descending from Col de la Rochette. The most diligent course recce wouldn't have unearthed a patch of tarmac softened by the midday sun, which sent Beloki skidding, breaking his femur, elbow and wrist. The organisers took notice and ever since 2003 now deploy water tankers before the peloton are due through, to spray sections of road that are susceptible to melting.

▽ Stricken Spaniard Joseph Beloki (centre) broke several bones at the 2003 Tour due to melting tarmac

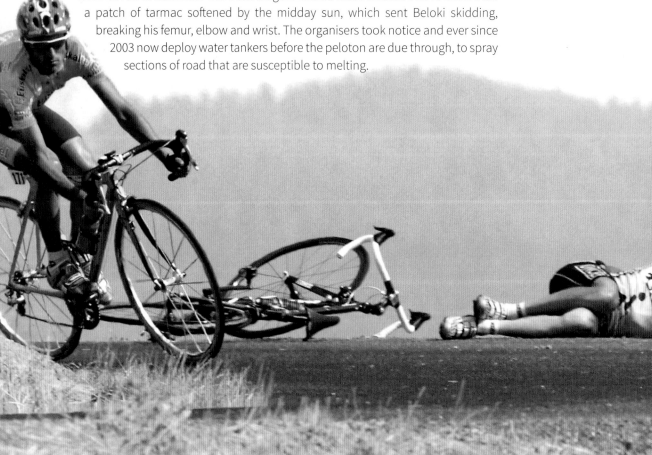

# REPLACING FLUIDS

On a six-hour hot stage, depending on what the rider's role or strategy is for the day, they can sweat up to 1.5 litres each hour. That adds up to nine litres over the course of the day, and as you're looking to lose no more than 2 per cent body weight, the ideal is that the rider will drink at least 8.82 litres during the race (one litre = one kilogram). As the Tour is a multi-stage race, hydration efforts begin the moment the rider wakes up.

'We visit the toilet and observe urine colour every morning of the Tour without fail,' says Michael Rogers of Tinkoff Sport. 'We have a colour chart to gauge how hydrated or dehydrated we are. If we're dehydrated, one of the simplest methods to hydrate is to sip cordial until the stage begins.'

Urine charts are the norm for most teams, as is weighing the riders, though Team Sky are a touch more high-tech and use a device that monitors dehydration from a urine sample. In fact, Rogers's idea stems from his days at Team Sky where they adhered to what they called 'a positive hydration strategy'. Simplified, that meant giving riders drinks all of the time rather than waiting for them to ask, but giving them drinks like pineapple juice over water as the nutritionists noted they'd leave half a glass of water and fail to drink enough. 'The last thing you want to do is wake up on day 15 and knock back a litre of water,' adds Rogers.

Urine charts are a simple way to measure hydration but don't come without their flaws. Rob Child, performance biochemist at Team Dimension Data, recalls the 2014 Vuelta, where temperatures tipped over 40°C in the shade.

'That was a crazy hot race,' he says. 'I always get feedback on the riders' hydration levels but it wasn't as simple as saying your urine is this colour so you're dehydrated. Take B vitamins, for example. They're heavily pigmented so a strong colour and give the riders' wee an orange hue. It's also difficult to tell between de-hydration and beetroot juice [see Chapter 3 for why beetroot juice is good] because both can elicit a darkish red tinge.'

Child explains that once he's distinguished whether it's the supplement or dehydration causing the darker wee, it's all about the window between breakfast and the stage start – which is around two hours, so there's still time to address

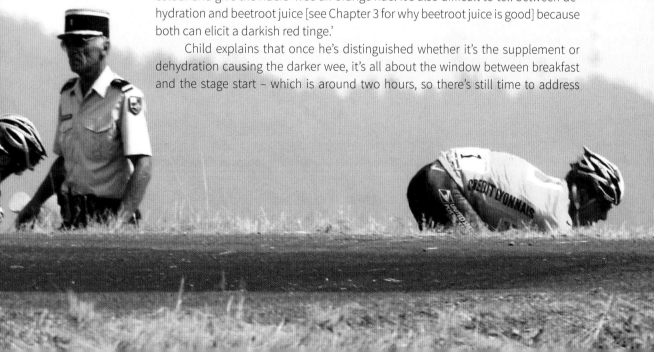

dehydration issues. 'As well as water, we might make them a couple of bespoke bottles on the bike (with added electrolytes, for instance) that could last a couple of hours, though perhaps more like 90 minutes in the heat.'

Individualised nutrition strategies are becoming more common at WorldTour level, though primarily before and after the stage. 'In a laboratory, you can give a subject almost anything you want to,' says Child. 'In a race, you have to compromise. At the feed zone [see 'What's a feed zone?' box below for more detail], for instance, you'll have nine guys and each might like a different drink, but there has to be compromise so we'll have probably two drinks to choose from. Those kind of compromises, you just don't think of them in a lab.'

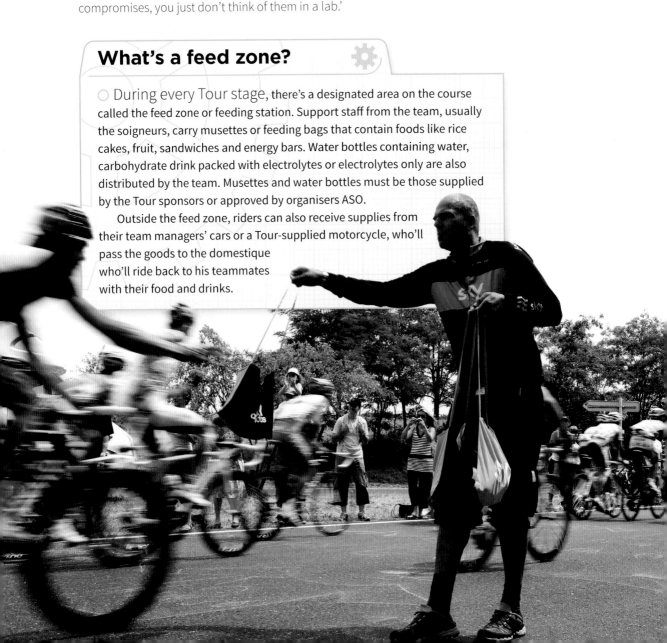

▽ Soigneur Maarten Mimpen hands out musettes to Team Sky riders

## What's a feed zone?

○ **During every Tour stage**, there's a designated area on the course called the feed zone or feeding station. Support staff from the team, usually the soigneurs, carry musettes or feeding bags that contain foods like rice cakes, fruit, sandwiches and energy bars. Water bottles containing water, carbohydrate drink packed with electrolytes or electrolytes only are also distributed by the team. Musettes and water bottles must be those supplied by the Tour sponsors or approved by organisers ASO.

Outside the feed zone, riders can also receive supplies from their team managers' cars or a Tour-supplied motorcycle, who'll pass the goods to the domestique who'll ride back to his teammates with their food and drinks.

The practical issues of custom-made nutrition strategies is highlighted further by Peter Hespel, nutritionist and coach at Etixx–Quick-Step. 'Having bottles made up for each and every rider would be a nightmare for soigneurs,' he says. 'In very heavy stages in the heat, soigneurs have to prepare 200 bidons. That's a hell of a job so it has to be a balance between tailor-made and practicality. Even at Team Sky, I'm sure while Froome would request a special composition, not all the riders would get one.'

Whichever the riders choose – bespoke or standard commercial bottles (like SiS, Powerbar and CNS) – they'll feature a number of electrolytes, including sodium. 'Normally the riders will have two bottles: one featuring electrolytes, water and carbohydrates, and one simply water,' says Josu Larrazabal, trainer at Trek-Segafredo. 'We try and keep that balance throughout every stage but it's not easy in the heat. The guys will come back to the car for bidons and we'll give them one of each. They'll say they just want water but you've still got to get electrolytes and carbs in.'

# SODIUM NEEDS

The most vital electrolyte for the sweating riders is sodium, which helps to maintain blood plasma volume and transport water from the bloodstream to working muscles. If the rider's drinks contained water with hardly any sodium, the body wouldn't retain it and it'd just be leached out into their soggy chamois.

Sweat contains sodium so the more you sweat, the more sodium you lose. But replacing these sodium losses isn't easy, as how much you sweat comes down to a number of different factors.

'One aspect that can play a role here is where a rider grew up,' explains Haudum. 'If you're, say, Australian, you can probably cope better with the heat than someone born and raised in Norway. You've adapted to it from an early age. But that's not the full story. Your body type will have an effect, too. Look at Cadel Evans. He was a rider who packed a lot of muscle mass, and if you have more muscle, that means you sweat more and lose more electrolytes. If you compared someone less muscular like Alberto, based on muscle mass I'd suspect that Cadel's more of a concern with dehydration than Contador.'

Andy Blow, a former elite triathlete, became so obsessed with the role sodium plays in hydration that in 2011 he launched a company called H2Pro Hydrate. H2Pro prescribe electrolyte tablets based on your sweat rate. Surprisingly the rider doesn't need to exercise to gain results. They simply tag a couple of electrodes that have been applied with polycarbonate onto the subject. That simulates the sweat glands. Blow then draws some sweat, puts it through a sweat analyser and discovers the composition of sweat in millimoles per litre. Blow and his team will then prescribe products ranging from 250mg of sodium a litre to 1,500mg.

'In the past we've done sweat tests for Garmin riders, the idea being they'd

 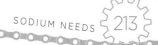

implement individual hydration plans,' explains Blow, though he concedes individualised race nutrition has practicality issues. 'It still makes sense, though – electrolyte composition in an individual can vary eight to tenfold person to person. Multiply that over 21 stages and you could find, if they haven't the right strategy, the heavy sweaters could have a disadvantage.'

Blow cites the example of Moto GP rider Eugene Laverty who had problems for years with fatigue and listlessness, especially during races in the heat. His sweat test showed that he lost 1,800g of sodium per litre, which is huge. Laverty's now playing around with sodium nutrition strategies to overcome this deficit. That means consuming high-salt foods like pretzels, which is a strategy used by many riders during a hot stage of the Tour.

'Tour riders shouldn't go the other way, though,' warns Blow. 'We tested Daniel Lloyd a few years back when he was racing for the Cervélo TestTeam because he'd actually gained weight during a Grand Tour. Because the race was hot, the nutritionist gave the riders more salt than normal. Broadly speaking, that's sensible advice, but Lloyd was a low sweater so retained electrolytes easily. The extra salt just retained more fluid, meaning extra weight.'

There are now a myriad of electrolyte tablets available to the rider, each with varying amounts of sodium, and each team will have hydration guidelines in place for each stage. But theory's one thing – in the heat, with fatigue rife, feel can dictate consumption more than regimen. 'We'll tend to have isotonic drinks [i.e. with similar concentrations of salt and sugar as in the human body], so they'll have less sugar,' says Koen de Kort, part of Giant-Alpecin's lead-out team. 'That's good because you're drinking so much, you don't want to make yourself sick. Despite everyone's best efforts, the idea's really to drink as much as you can stomach but you'll still be dehydrated at the end!'

Part of that struggle simply boils down to practicality. When you're cruising on the flats, chatting to the rider next to you, taking regular sips from your water bottle is as natural and easy as breathing. But as the intensity rises, things change. 'On the big mountain stages, you'd want to plan it that the last half-hour of the climb you're hardly touching the fluids,' says Rogers. 'That means taking on a lot more fluid in the less-intense parts of the stage.'

On crossing the line of a hot stage, riders will continue to sip and drink electrolytes, the aim not only to replenish fluids from the stage but in preparation for the following day's effort. And then it's back to the team hotel? Not quite, if you've had a good day.

'It's harder to follow certain recovery protocols if you're successful as you'll have to visit doping control,' says Haudum. 'If you're pretty dehydrated, it can take over an hour.' The race leader and stage winner are tested, as are six to eight riders selected at random. A specially equipped caravan is based near the finish line of every stage to transport drug samples to a private location following the race. Drug

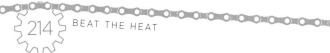

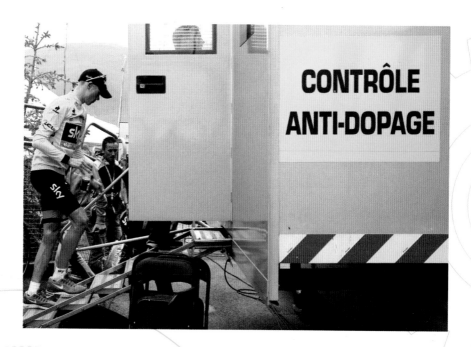

## CHAPTER 11

▷ Doping control can take over an hour if a rider is suffering from dehydration

test samples are then transported by private plane for analysis and results are quickly reported to Tour officials. Michel Pollentier was clearly in a hurry at the 1978 Tour. After winning the Alpe d'Huez stage, he was caught with someone else's urine in a rubber bulb tucked into his bib shorts. He was ejected from the Tour. Ironically, his real urine tested negative!

So you've finished the stage – how do the teams make sure their riders hydrate as quickly as possible? Team Dimension Data's performance biochemist Rob Child uses a technique applied on the Asian continent for thousands of years. 'If it's a particularly hot stage and I see that the whole team's dehydrated, I'll modify what I'm cooking and add more spices. That tends to increase the riders' thirst and encourages them to keep drinking.'

Like all areas of performance at the Tour de France, hydration is an evolving field. While the teams aim for no more than those 2 per cent body weight losses through the stage, recent research from Brock University scientist and avid cyclist Stephen Cheung suggests this figure isn't set in stone.

'My studies showed that a loss of 3 per cent or so wouldn't impact as much as you'd think it would, or as much as you're told it would,' says Cheung. 'It might increase your heart rate a little bit – which we showed – and increase your core temperature a bit but none of our subjects reached any critical levels. Yes, it was physically more stressful but didn't impact on performance.'

Cheung's research is supported by a paper in the *British Journal of Sports Medicine* entitled, 'Current hydration guidelines are erroneous: dehydration does

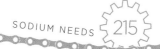

not impair performance in the heat'. The researchers showed that when well-trained cyclists performed a 25km time trial in the heat, while it showed rectal temperature (not to be taken on the Tour!) was higher beyond 17km of the time trial, no other differences were observed.

A further study from France weighed 643 runners before and after a marathon and showed that the fastest runners lost the most fluid weight on average; the slowest runners kept their losses below 2 per cent. Running legend Haile Gebrselassie has been shown to lose as much as 10 per cent of his starting weight while running marathons – and still managed to set two world records.

But where the Tour differs is its multi-stage element. All of this research focused on one-off bouts of exercise. At the Tour, you have 21 bouts and that de-hydration would add up. You suspect 2 per cent will remain the target for the foreseeable future.

## WHAT TO WEAR IN THE HEAT

In 2014, to welcome in the New Year, Team Sky's Chris Froome tweeted a picture of his and his team's new skinsuit. 'This skin suit takes #marginalgains to the next level,' it read. Many suggested it should have had a 9pm watershed rating as the mesh skinsuit left little to the imagination. 'Yes they're revealing,' says Team Sky's Luke Rowe, who competed at his first Tour de France in 2015. 'But deal with it. Man up.'

You can see why a mesh suit would improve cooling – greater airflow sweeping over the skin, promoting a higher level of evaporative cooling. 'It certainly cools but it's not great from a UV protection standpoint,' explains Simon Huntsman, head of R&D at Rapha. 'If the riders do choose to go with the mesh suit or top, they must lather up with loads of suncream.'

Rapha is a London-born apparel brand that began supplying clothes to Team Sky in 2013. They're known for their aesthetically pleasing performance wear married with intelligent use of innovative materials. While the mesh suit grabbed the headlines, it's their – and other manufacturers like Tinkoff Sport apparel supplier Sportful's – use of so-called cooling fabrics that provides an extra, albeit thin, layer of protection.

'When it's hot, it's all about heat management and keeping the rider comfortable,' says Huntsman. 'Managing that heat effectively is always tricky in high summer but we use a number of different technology platforms to try and improve cooling.'

'The first one is the weight of the garments,' he continues. 'Weight will affect comfort so we try and keep the tops as light as we can without compromising the integrity. We also look at the structure of the textiles because when the rider is moving, he's created a dynamic environment.'

Enter wicking. This is the process where moisture is drawn away from the skin and, in this case, to the surface of the cycle top. Because water conducts heat more than 20 times quicker than air, if sweat is left to pool on the skin, your skin temperature rises, which would ultimately lead to a drop in performance. 'That's why one of the

▷ Cyril Lemoine of Cofidis collects water bottles from the team car for his fellow riders

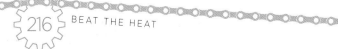

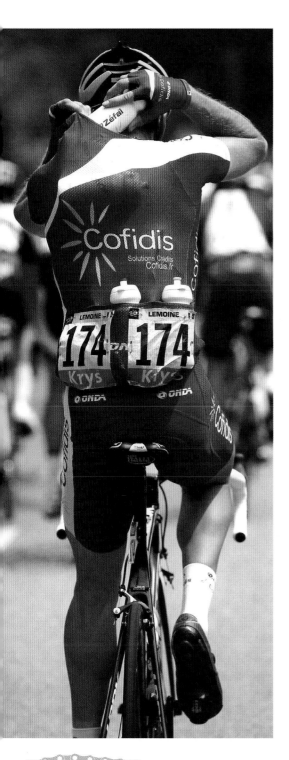

key challenges to keeping comfortable is to reduce the amount of water that sits on the surface or in the fabric. Evaporated cooling is a constant target,' says Huntsman.

In intense heat, no fabric can currently provide the ideal evaporative cooling system to wick and dry in an instant. But there are technologies out there that give it a damn good try. Team Sky use a performance polyester yarn called Coolmax, a cross-section of which resembles a big flower. The idea is that the greater the surface area, the more effective a garment is at moving moisture down the yarn and into the atmosphere.

You'd think colour choice would be a heat-management imperative, too. Elementary physics states that black absorbs all wavelengths of light and converts them into heat, while a white object reflects all wavelengths of light so the light isn't converted to heat and the temperature of the object doesn't noticeably rise. That's why you can clearly see Tour teams wearing lighter colours like Tinkoff (yellow), Katusha (white) and FDJ (equally white).

'Yes, one of the challenges of designing Sky's kit is the colour, namely black,' says Huntsman. 'There's obviously a potential of absorbency. So that's why we use a technology called Coldblack.'

Coldblack is a textile finish developed by Swiss company Schoeller that reflects both visible and invisible rays of sunlight, showing up to a 5°C drop over non-treated black tops. 'Ultimately that means less fatigue,' says Huntsman.

Rapha are experts at providing fit and selecting suitable fabrics for the job. They're now looking to create their own fabrics rather than rely on outside suppliers – which is exactly what Michael Rogers managed at the 2014 Tour when he invented the BAR jersey. The mesh top is slipped on by the domestique who can then load it with water bottles for his thirsty teammates. It's a simple solution to the age-old problem of the dutiful domestique carrying bottles from the team car and offloading them to his team. Rogers was well qualified to design a hydration solution – he has form in this area …

# SLUSH PUPPIE SOLUTION

In the build-up to the Beijing Olympics in 2008, sports scientists from national federations around the globe had one major issue to contend with: how to manage the intense heat and humidity. One of the most forward-thinking was the Australian Institute of Sport (AIS), hoping to help Rogers and Cadel Evans with their ambitions of claiming gold in the individual time trial.

'We spent a lot of time in the lab with physiologists like Louis Burke,' says Rogers, 'and most of it was around lowering core body temperature in the heat. I just remember swallowing a big pill that measured core temperature at different intensities.'

The research was much more involved than that. The team at the AIS recruited 12 top-level cyclists and began trialling new methods to reduce their core temperature. After much experimentation, they discovered that athletes drinking 700–1,000ml of an ice slushie made by Gatorade realised a drop of 0.5°C. After a 30-minute warm-up, that 0.5°C reduction remained. The researchers also wrapped

▽ Koen de Kort consumes ice slushie with the aim of reducing core temperature

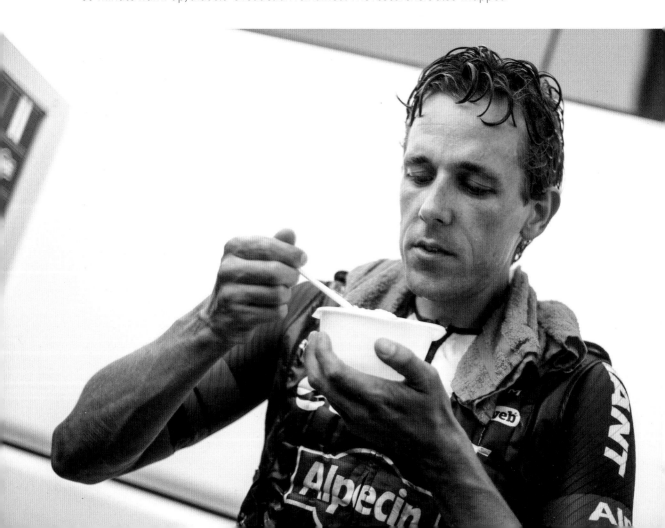

cold towels around the rider's legs and body but, despite showing positive results in their trial, this was thought to negate the benefits of the warm-up: it cooled down the muscles the athletes were looking to warm.

Burke also added glycerol to the slushie to improve fluid retention as studies had shown that consuming glycerol could retain up to 50 per cent more fluid than water alone. The UCI were convinced of its merits and banned the use of glycerol in 2010 due to its 'plasma-expanding' qualities.

The results of the study were startling with an average 66-second improvement over 40km, so the team applied the strategy in Beijing. As it transpired, Rogers missed out on the gold medal, finishing eighth; Evans finished fifth. And the idea seemed to die a death… until the 2014 Tour de France. While Marcel Kittel and John Degenkolb warmed up for the time trial, slushing away in the background was a machine that looked mightily like a Slush Puppie machine.

'It *was* a Slush Puppie machine,' says Teun van Erp, sports scientist at Giant-Alpecin. 'I picked up and adapted the idea from AIS research because my studies showed it's well worth using. We tested it at training camps before the Tour and the riders were really enthusiastic about it. They felt it helped them push more power in the heat.'

Teun observed that the riders' bodies could store heat for longer because of the reduced baseline temperature. While your body starts to close down when internal temperatures get up near 39.5°C, the cooler your core is to begin with, the more thermal legroom you have to ride hard. 'We noticed a positive effect on performance of 3–8 per cent depending on the cooling, the person and the environment though we'd only really used Slush Puppie when over 25°C', says van Erp. 'It's also more useful for shorter, more intense stages like time trials.'

Just to add some carbohydrate topping to the slushie cake, the ice mixture also included a 2:1 ratio of glucose to fructose. On paper it certainly looks like a rather palatable way to begin an hour of eyes-out cycling; in practice, the reality is slightly more painful. 'It really cools your core but the problem is, you can't just eat it and enjoy it,' says de Kort. 'To avoid it melting and warming up, you basically have to swallow the ice without swilling it around in your mouth. This could upset your stomach. So far, though, I've been okay.'

Research has also shown that consuming an ice slushie after a stage can help recovery. That got Team Dimension Data's performance biochemist Rob Child thinking. 'Often the weather conditions will dictate what I serve up on the bus after a stage. I was in Portugal with the team and it was a particularly hot day, so I thought they might like some ice slushie. Then I thought how useful it would be to pack in some slow-releasing carbohydrates and protein, too. So I thought why not make some rice pudding, add a sprinkle of protein powder and stick it in the freezer. It lowered core, refuelled and repaired muscle all in one go. But, more importantly, they liked it.'

# How a rider loses heat

○ Core body temperature is around 37°C. During high-intensity exercise in a hot environment, this can easily rise above 38°C, leading to a performance decline and potential muscle cramps.

Around 40°C and the rider could be crippled by heat exhaustion, leading to nausea and headaches. Over 40°C and heatstroke's a real concern. Symptoms include confusion, nausea and visual problems. Immediate medical attention is needed to prevent brain damage, organ failure or even death. Thankfully, there are four key ways the Tour rider loses heat from their exercising body to maintain a stable core temperature: radiation, evaporation, convection and conduction.

**Convection:** This is the process of losing heat through the movement of air or water molecules across the skin. It's why increased wind speed through faster pedalling increases wind-chill.

**Evaporation:** Process of losing heat through the conversion of water to gas; in other words, the evaporation of sweat.

Solar radiation

**Radiation:** The heat generated from within the body and given off to the atmosphere in the form of infrared rays. Involves the transfer of heat from one object to another with no physical contact involved.

**Conduction:** Where you lose heat through physical contact with another object. If your saddle was cooler than your buttocks, heat would flow to your saddle.

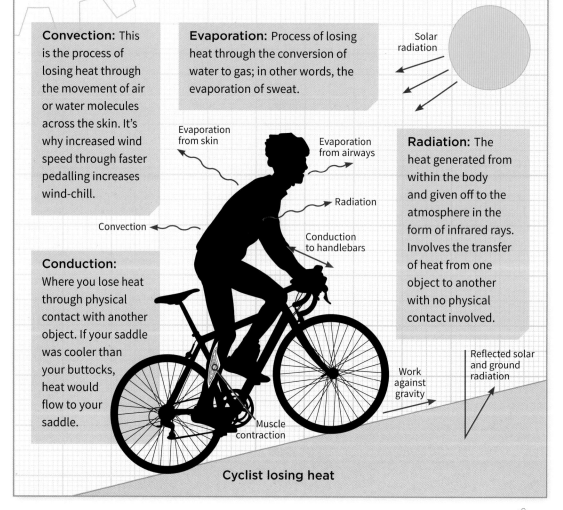

Evaporation from skin

Evaporation from airways

Radiation

Convection

Conduction to handlebars

Muscle contraction

Work against gravity

Reflected solar and ground radiation

**Cyclist losing heat**

▽ Ice vests are a
common sight at
the Tour de France

# VESTS AND TIGHTS

Another cooling innovation that Team Dimension Data, Giant-Alpecin and a number of teams have adopted from the Olympics is the ice vest. This concept stretches back to the 1996 Atlanta Games where Australian rowers stuffed ice packs into their vests during the warm-up. Now it's unusual for a rider to be warming up on the turbo for a hot stage not to be wearing this cooling apparel.

'I wear a cooling vest before the start of a time trial or an important stage,' says de Kort. 'I wear it for about 20 minutes – usually when I'm warming up on the rollers.' That's despite much research showing very few actual cooling benefits. 'We only use them between 20–25°C,' says van Erp, 'and they're not as beneficial as ice drinks.' It's a view echoed by Larrazabal at Trek. 'Yes, we use them as they cool down the skin and create a nice feeling. However, they don't really cool down the core so it's more a sensory impact than a physiological one.'

That feeling of pleasure leads to another WorldTour confession: as soon as the mercury rises, Froome and co. love to press women's tights against their flesh. 'Like many teams, we use ice socks down the back of our necks,' says Rowe. 'All you do is get a woman's stocking, fill it with ice, cut it in sections and stick it down the back of your neck. They really help.'

Michael Rogers agrees, rating it the number-one strategy out of all the ice-cooling practices employed by Tinkoff Sport. You'll find every team car has a freezer nestled in the boot. Within lies enough ice to build an igloo and enough tights to clothe a catwalk. Look closely

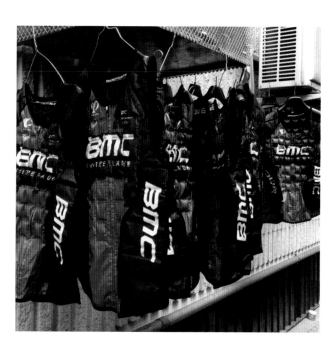

around the streets of France in July and you'll no doubt come across a discarded pair of pantyhose once stuffed down Andrew Talansky's cycle shirt. Or, in the case of Trek-Segafredo and Messrs Mollema and Cancellara, wristbands.

'During a hot stage, we have one guy come back for the bottles and one for the wristbands,' says Larrazabal. 'They're wristbands that are sprayed with ice liquid and kept in the cooling box. They then either put it over their hands or wrists for some cooling relief.'

'When the guys pick up the bottles and bands, we also throw the liquid over their body, legs and head,' he adds. 'It gives them a feeling of freshness.' Like the ice vests and tights,

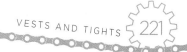

the liquid doesn't remain cool long to significantly impact core temperature, but the psychological boost is enough to maintain power output. Recent research from South Africa and Australia suggests that athletes may subconsciously select a pace based on psychological perceptions of heat stress; in other words, those riders who perceive they have a hotter brain will perform slower.

That ice-based theme continues post-stage. How to cool down effectively and aid recovery? Many teams still offer the traditional ice bath – despite recent research suggesting its use may blunt muscular adaptation (see Chapter 10 for more) – though teams with healthier budgets may also employ the iCool system.

'We still use it a little bit for cooling,' says Brent Bookwalter, domestique at BMC Racing. 'Basically you sit in an inflatable pool and it circulates cold water. BMC has a spare van and there are a couple of them set up in there. One of the team is in charge of driving this to each hotel and setting it up. We'll come out of the bus after a transfer, and if core temperature is still up after a hot stage, we'll get in. You stay in for around 10–15 minutes.'

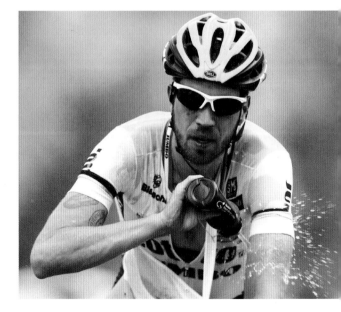

▽ Cool water is a good psychological tactic to cope with the heat, as seen by Lotto NL – Jumbo cyclist Martijn Keizer at the 2016 Tour Down Under in Australia

# HEAT ACCLIMATION

Preparing for the heat – or heat acclimation – is another string in the rider's heat-related bow. Simply put, the rider spends a certain period of time in the heat to stimulate a series of physiological changes that'll prepare them for the extra demands of racing in this extreme environment. Research has shown that healthy adults exposed to conditions that elevate their core temperature by 1°C to 2°C for 60–90 minutes over a period of four to ten days will afterwards elicit a lower resting core temperature, greater blood plasma volume and an increased sweating rate – all favourable adaptations to exercising in the heat.

Tales of riders sitting in saunas to acclimatise stretch back to the early 20th century, but one of the most extreme methods took place in Liverpool, England, in the 1990s. Chris Boardman, who set the record for the fastest average speed recorded in a Tour stage of 55.2km/h in 1994 (before BMC Racing's Rohan Dennis raised the record to 55.446km/h at the 2015 Tour's prologue in Utrecht), would often turbo train in a bedroom in his English home with a radiator cranking out the heat. Just for good measure, the window frames were sealed with tape to avoid cooling draughts.

It's a technique that could have benefited Welshman Luke Rowe in 2013.

'I remember the Tour of California and a couple of the days were in the low to mid-40s,' he says. 'You're out there in the middle of the desert and there's no hiding place. That was especially true for me as I was riding out front in support of Bradley Wiggins. It was a stark change to racing the Tour of Romandie just a couple weeks before where the stages were shortened because of snow!'

In truth, antics like Boardman's when he was training for the Olympics are rarer in road racing where the riders either live (Nairo Quintana) or have second homes (Cavendish in Girona) in locations that are hot all-year round. There's also the racing that starts in January at the Tour Down Under, taking place during an Australian summer, and is followed in February by races in the UAE before temperatures plummet for the spring classics.

'You find that once the classics are over, heat acclimation kind of happens in a progressive way,' says Larrazabal. 'Many of the guys at Trek live and train in Spain but they'll also race California, the Dauphiné or Switzerland – all of which prepare them for the Tour.'

There's also the thermal-management that derives from being incredibly fit. Similar to heat acclimation, as your fitness grows, you experience a host of adaptations that are naturally conducive to racing fast in the heat. These include an improved sweat response to dissipate heat quickly, which stems from both lower core temperature thresholds for the initiation of sweating and greater sensitivity of sweating response to increasing core temperature.

'Improved aerobic capacity also leads to elevated plasma volume and cardiac output,' says Brock University's Stephen Cheung. 'This minimises the competition for blood distribution between skeletal muscle and skin.' In short, as Sagan, Nibali and Valverde rack up the miles, their bodies develop a greater capacity for, and a slower rate of, heat storage.

Still, despite professional cyclists' physiological adaptation to the heat, they are only human. A scan of the Rodez finish line at the 13th stage of the 2015 Tour, where temperatures tipped past 40°C, resembled a desert war scene with exhausted riders held upright by their loyal soigneurs. 'There's going to be a world shortage of bottles after this race, I reckon,' joked Cannondale-Garmin's Dan Martin, who's moved to Etixx–Quick-Step for the 2016 season. Teammate Nathan Haas reflected the day's events more poetically. 'It's atrotious,' he said. 'It's something you can't describe; the feeling that when the heat goes so deep within you, it feels like it's in your bones.' But the scientists continue to research new nutrition, training and equipment protocols to retain a core temperature that'll deliver optimum performance. Researchers and manufacturers are also creating tools and techniques that could redefine the cycling landscape, sending the riders ever faster to Paris. And emerging technologies is where we head next.

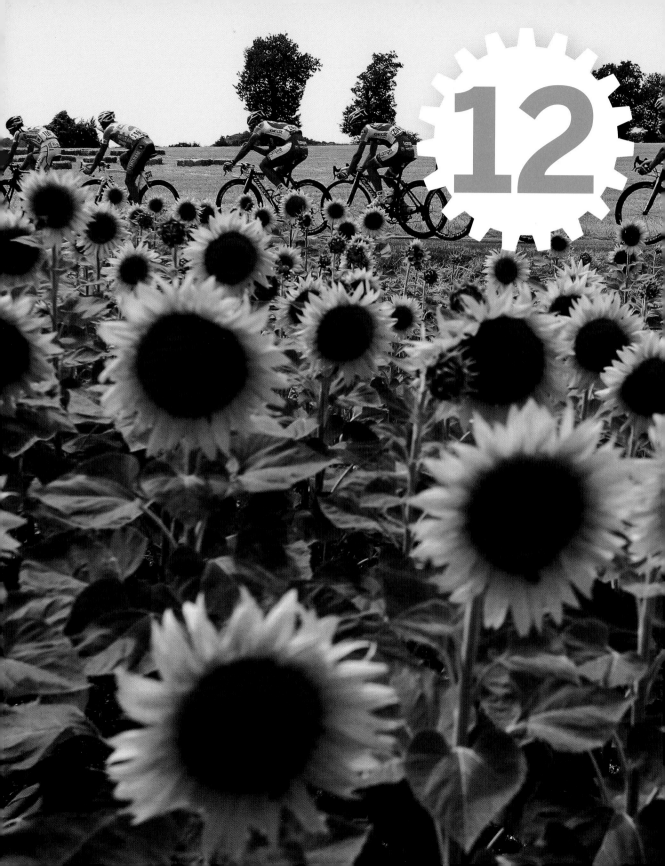

12

# MARGINAL GAINS 2.0

At the start of 2015, Dave Brailsford flew to San Francisco with Team Sky's data scientist Robby Ketchell. The visit attracted headlines because Brailsford visited 20 tech companies in search of the next big thing – or things – that could help his riders go faster. At one point on his visit, Brailsford was pictured with electrodes attached to his head while playing darts. 'It's a form of cranial stimulation,' he told the *Guardian*'s Sean Ingle. 'The military have been using it for their snipers to reduce the time it takes them to acquire a skill. What they are suggesting is that this increases the plasticity of the cortex to enable fast-track leaning. After a while they sent an electric current to see whether it could improve my play.'

And it worked – 'I went from shit to less shit,' Brailsford said laughing. You won't see Froome and Porte connected to the national grid while ascending the Galibier anytime soon, though wearable technologies and apps will become more prevalent across the board. 'Muscle Sound is one to keep an eye on,' says Ketchell. 'They non-invasively measure glycogen content, which would obviously help with aspects like training intensity and nutrition strategies.'

Ketchell says the numerous start-ups that populate San Francisco are a good place to uncover where the future of cycling lies. But why spend money on a plane ticket when you can simply ask industry insiders and riders what gear, training or nutritional development will have the greatest impact on professional cycling?

◁ The peloton rides past sunflower fields from Rodez to Revel

## CHRIS BOARDMAN ✱ TOUR DE FRANCE PROLOGUE WINNER, 1994

'**When it comes to wind tunnels,** the cycling industry has moved from not knowing that there's something they don't know, to knowing there's something they don't know. No one's really got to grips with an ongoing strategy of understanding. People here and there are using wind tunnels, and trying to develop ways to measure aerodynamics, but no one has a strategic way to consistently look at the greatest user of energy.

'That's why I've just invested in a wind tunnel that's a third built, which you'll be able to use for aerodynamics, physiological testing, bike-fitting … it's a whole performance centre that'll cost not much more than the price of a curry to use.

'It'll be good for the pros, systematically teaching them why aerodynamics matters so much and how important it is; why it's worth exploring clothing and different positions. It has to be part of your standard training to fundamentally understand what's happening on a daily basis in a sport that's governed by aerodynamics. I want it to be as frequent as benchmark training sessions that the pros can nip into the wind tunnel and see how their coefficient of drag is changing. Affordable wind tunnel testing is the future.'

## PAUL LEW ✱ DIRECTOR OF INNOVATION AT REYNOLDS CYCLING

'**Disc brakes are being tested** in the professional peloton right now and, if all goes well, the UCI will allow them into the WorldTour from 2017. And that's a double-edged sword. On one hand, disc brakes have presented the biggest aerodynamic liability that wheel and frame manufacturers have had to overcome. But they've also presented the greatest opportunity to reshape bicycles and rim profiles to optimise aerodynamics. There are all kinds of new opportunities when the designer isn't restricted by the addition of a rim caliper. It's a great challenge with great rewards.

'It's a challenge for both wheel and frame manufacturers because both parties can innovate so much that it creates compatibility issues with fit and components, so innovations have to come in phases and steps. For instance, I can manufacture a wheel that might have outstanding dynamic performance because of a very innovative shape but it won't fit in a bike frame. Even when you remove the calipers, the fork and stays might be too narrow. Or the hub mount isn't optimised for width and dimension, so all this has to be taken into account.

'Innovation is a combination of wheel and bike manufacturer working together, and good communication between the two parties. I have some unique wheel ideas but they have to be within the boundaries of what's compatible with bike frame design.

'It's a strange one with disc brakes because their development has been driven by the masses where they're already available. I'm sure that once the UCI ratify them for professionals they'll prove popular. Mind you, if the UCI decide to reduce the minimum weight regulation, we might see a resurgence in high-end rim brake designs.

'This could result in exciting race situations where you see cyclists swapping bikes in the middle of a stage. You might see the 10–12 GC riders changing bikes multiple times so that they can descend at the fastest speed with a disc-brake bike and ascend at top speed with the super-light caliper brakes.'

## DR JONATHAN BAKER ✱ SPORTS SCIENTIST, TEAM DIMENSION DATA

'**This sounds vast** but we're keen to understand much more about the physiological stress imposed by a three-week Grand Tour. That's why we're looking to undertake research studies with the team at the Tour. We've done it at the Vuelta and it's a beneficial exercise. You collect data on numerous physiological components like exactly how much food they're eating; their body mass; how their hormonal profiles fluctuate after each and every stage. We'll look to publish the results in a research paper.

'Clearly we have to get the riders to buy into it, but if we can make it clear to them that they'll be learning things no one else knows – undertaking a real-life science experiment that'll benefit their performance – I'm sure they'll be keen.'

## JONATHAN VAUGHTERS ✱ TEAM MANAGER CANNONDALE-GARMIN

'**The most interesting thing** that I've seen is that people are poking around with a wearable monitor that determines lactate concentration in your bloodstream.

'For me, that's the next big shift in physiology because when you cross-correlate that information with heart rate and power data, you create a deeper, more rounded picture of what's happening to the rider; you begin to see metabolic triangulation. It'll tell you how hard the engine's working, how much power it's producing and what the by-products are of that effort.

'The brain's also an area of interest. I've noted some interesting research looking at hypoxia [oxygen deficiency] on the brain. Studies have shown that as circulation rises, so do intelligence levels, which go up and up and up with increasing effort until you reach a certain intensity and duration. That's when blood almost drops out of the brain. The blood flow to the brain significantly decreases within a certain timeframe, and is the precursor to your body saying, "No, we're not doing this anymore, we're slowing down." Hypoxic training could train these levels to a higher level – though how interested the riders would be in being oxygen-starved is a different matter.

'But sometimes you just have to make the leap from theory into application. Numerous studies have shown that X, Y and Z works well for an amateur athlete. That doesn't mean it'll work for the professional rider. One of the problems with academic research is that professional riders just don't have enough time on their hands to partake in these studies. There have been many avenues we've pursued down the years and it's just not worked. It's something you have to be aware of when chasing new technologies.'

## TEUN VAN ERP ✱ GIANT-ALPECIN SPORTS SCIENTIST

'**We're working on a device** where we can measure how much vibration there is within a bike. We're currently doing tests, and still have to work things out with the company we're collaborating with. We can also test things like tyres. Usually we say if tyres are wider, there's less vibration. With this we can measure that.

'We're also working on a project tied in with the anaerobic threshold of riders. Again, we did some tests and the results are pretty scientific but we still need to work it out. Cycling is becoming more scientific.'

## SAMUELE MARCORA ✳ PROFESSOR OF EXERCISE PHYSIOLOGY, UNIVERSITY OF KENT, ENGLAND

'**My psychobiological model** of fatigue suggests that it's not the physical or a subconscious message that stops us but our perception of fatigue. I had 10 male athletes perform a simple exercise protocol on stationary bikes. They rode as hard as they could for five seconds. The subjects then rode at a fixed power output until they could no longer sustain this wattage – or around 12 minutes on average – before repeating the five-second max test.

'I discovered that power output from the second max test was roughly 30 per cent lower than the first, but was still three times greater than the power generated when riding to exhaustion. So how could the subjects hardly pedal in creating 242 watts, before powering to 731 watts?

'It's down to motivation, which impacts perception of effort. When the effort is perceived as maximal or when the effort required eclipses the amount of effort you're willing to exert, you stop.

'The psychobiological model is a conscious awareness of the central motor command (brain and neural system), which sends signals to the active muscles and ties in with the physical models. If you have weaker muscles, you have to increase the activity of central motor command to compensate. This is perceived as in increase in effort and will stop you. Signs of "weaker muscles" are physical aspects like lower glycogen levels or acidosis. However, they have an indirect impact rather than directly stopping you. It's why caffeine is used. It's been shown to lower the perception of effort.

'There are simple cerebral activities designed to reduce your perception of effort. The first focuses on subliminal messages. These affect your subconscious brain and are based on cognitive science. In one study, I showed that positive words like "go", "energy" and "lively" motivated the group more than negative words like "stop", "toil" or "sleep", extending their workout time by 17 per cent.

'Then there's brain endurance training, a project I've received a grant from the Ministry of Defence to develop. Key is "response inhibition", which works in an area of the brain called the anterior cingulate cortex (ACC) and is linked to motivation and effort.

'I showed that by stimulating an athlete's ACC three times a week, focusing on something they don't like, athletes perceive less fatigue. My team are currently working on apps that'll tap into this area. My model is about endurance performance and what role your mind plays in the physical outcome.'

## STEVE SMITH ✳ BRAND MANAGER AT SPORTFUL

'**We've looked at a lot of stuff,** including integrating heart-rate sensors into clothing.

'We've also looked at temperature sensors, but the problem is that in integrating these bits of technology, we have to make a heavier garment. Right now there are still some big gains to be had from aerodynamics.

'Helping the rider to ride at optimal temperature is also a big deal. It's pretty natural that when you jump on your bike, after half an hour of riding, your core temperature might have increased by 1°C but that's normal. If your body heats up by another 0.5°C, performance will drop dramatically. And that makes sense. If you have a fever, you're just laying in bed and feel terrible. So if you had a fever on the bike, you'd feel terrible. So we're continuing to look at methods to innovate wicking and cooling.'

# DAVID MARTIN ✻ EXERCISE PHYSIOLOGIST AT THE AUSTRALIAN INSTITUTE OF SPORT

'**MIT has developed something** called a sociometer and I think this could have a role to play in the future of team sports like cycling. It's a complicated one but let me explain …

'Because humans are complicated and are social and have emotions, there's a really difficult overlay of sad athletes and angry athletes, happy athletes and bored athletes, and motivated athletes. Which is a pain in the butt because, as a coach, we know that these athletes are so fit, they could win any race. But they don't for a variety of reasons.

'You'll hear a lot of athletes say "I won this gold medal and would like to thank my coach because he believed in me". They'll say, "I am just part of a great team. We have a shared vision and I love my team". What the sociometer is doing is trying to put metrics behind those concepts.

'The basic idea behind a sociometer is that you and I are connecting right now. And there'll be a whole bunch of people in your life that connect with you. There is this idea of human and verbal communication that strengthens connectivity in groups. So you can start to build up these diagrams, of ball and stick figures, that look like clouds of connectivity.

'You begin to see every person as a node and every link is based on communication. If you are a small dot and only have one thin line coming to you, it means you're not really connecting with anyone. If you're a big dot, it means lots of people connect with you. If it's a big thick line, it means you're in constant conversation and dialogue with other nodes (or people).

'As you communicate with people a lot, you start to draw those nodes closer and closer to your node. If you don't communicate very often or very long, people start to separate away from you. So what you get is these really interesting diagrams

that paint a picture of organisation that shows this individual is connected to the team.

'It pulses and has a timeframe to it. There are times when you're really connected; sometimes not connected. In the future, I think we'll see blueprints that are very healthy and conducive to world-class performances. We'll also see social environment diagrams that aren't good at all. And see stuff in the middle.

'The magic of the future is not only to observe decaying communication or links but to actually do something about it. To include the individuals who are a catalyst for the positive change you're after within a group. Getting the timing right and remedying alien relationships.

'I think we all feel it; we feel the confidence wane from a team. We feel the general morale drop. Some individuals are intuitively good at making a light joke or trying to improve the situation. Some coaches are phenomenal leaders who have a great ability to connect and reposition the team. This is interesting feedback for teams to say that there's technology out there that will help the team move in a positive direction. It's a blend of neurophysiology, organisation psychology and sports science.

'Practically, there are some easy applications. The rider spends a lot of time on their bike. All I have to do is wire up the bike with a directional microphone and a proximity detector. I'll be able to tell if someone chats to someone else and where they are in position to each other. Over a six-hour ride, you might get a fingerprint of the team's dynamic. They wouldn't even need to know. You could just say, "in this team we ride these bikes and they're instrumented in a number of different ways". Cyclists are masters of modelling.'

 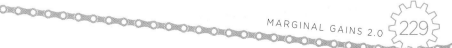

## JAMIE PRINGLE ✷
### EXERCISE PHYSIOLOGIST AT THE ENGLISH INSTITUTE OF SPORT

'**Training in the morning** is often cited as the preferable time of the day to train as testosterone levels show a circadian decline from when you wake. Strength training in the morning could also elicit greater rewards later on. 'My colleague, Liam Kilduff, showed that morning exercise primes the body for afternoon competition. A short, high-force workout early on that taxes the entire kinetic chain, like a back squat, stimulates a favourable testosterone response in the afternoon. We've used this strategy at British Cycling for afternoon competition and it's a good primer for peak performance.'

## CHRIS YU ✷
### AERODYNAMICS ENGINEER AT SPECIALIZED

'**Where we stand to gain** is by custom building things. One example is having a more dynamic simulator, like you'd have in Formula One. They can simulate their entire race in the wind tunnel from different approaches and speeds.

'We have a projector built into our wind tunnel. Imagine if we load up a time-trial course on video and you're riding that in the wind tunnel, with twists and turns into crosswinds and out of crosswinds, utilising turntable dials that helps to mimic the course and wind profile. That's somewhere we can and will go.'

## TIM LAWSON ✷ HEAD OF NUTRITION COMPANY 'SECRET TRAINING'

'**When I sold Science in Sport** [UK nutrition company], the patent for GoGel went with it. We needed a new process, not just a new formulation. Luckily when researching the area of preserving and improving the bioavailability of fish oils with my new company Secret Training, I stumbled across some research that showed there might be an interesting way to process rice starch. Sticky rice starch has great absorption characteristics. It also means that we could include fructose in the solution so you enjoy the benefit of multiple transporters [see page 173]. It's based on unique technology for creating gels. We've had a few interesting experiments along the way. We pushed the technology a touch too far and basically had a bar in a wrapper because the gels were hardening up. The starch can retrograde very quickly, and it's worse if you put it in the fridge. But it's ready – and we're always looking for margins.'

## STEPHEN CHEUNG ✷ PROFESSOR OF ERGONOMICS, BROCK UNIVERSITY, CANADA

'**There's a lot of work** examining the psychology of exercise that feeds into exercise regulation. A researcher in Wales did a nice study examining how quickly you pick up a mental template for exercise intensity. He had two groups. One was told they were going to do a 4km effort four times a day with breaks. They knew what they were going to do and they were getting full feedback. The experimental group was told that they were also doing four efforts and that they were identical in length but they weren't told what that length was. Also, they weren't given any feedback during the trial. With the full knowledge group, performance was dead flat. The experimental group started way up here but by the third effort, wham – dovetailed right in like the other group. That study tells me how quickly you set this mental template of whatever the distance, even without power meters and speedometers, you instantly resume perfect pace.

'Mental training is still a fledgling field but if you can tap into areas like raising this pacing template, performance gains could be huge.'

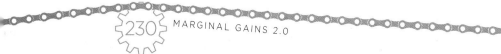

# CONCLUSION

Genetics will also play an important role in training and identifying champions. 'I know of teams who have had DNA testing,' says Tinkoff Sport's head of sport science Daniel Healey. 'I've seen data and I believe there is a place for it.' The idea is that the sports scientist could examine a rider's genetic make-up and ensure that their current role in the team is genetically suitable. If the test reveals that genetic providence has blessed them with huge amounts of endurance and the rider's a sprinter, it might be worth a rethink of their position in the team. Though telling someone like Peter Sagan that their DNA report means they're now to be trained as a domestique could be an awkward conversation. Realistically, the genetic report might throw up details about potential injury risk or recovery rate, which could be fed back into their training.

Where genetics could play a greater role in the evolution of professional cycling is in the hands of Yannis Pitsiladis, professor of sport and exercise science at Brighton University, England. Pitsiladis is working on a test that detects doping by uncovering each drug's genetic fingerprint. While a drug is taking effect, thousands of tiny molecules called mRNA transcribe instructions for constructing the proteins that bring about physiological changes. Pitsiladis's work with the gene technology known as 'omics' detects this genetic activity rather than, in the case of doping, blood volume and blood cells. It also has the potential to uncover micro-doping.

'This is the cutting-edge of anti-doping,' says Pitsiladis.

Genetics clearly has a role to play in refining training practices and keeping the sport clean. Aerodynamics, nutrition and wearable technologies will all be refined, albeit how much they'll be applied at races is down to the UCI.

The brain will also become an even greater focal point of research. With theories like Marcora's and Tim Noakes's celebrated central governor model of fatigue, there's a great appetite to break down perceived physical barriers where the human potentially constructs them – in the brain. But this area needs a credible and significant breakthrough, and that means, as Jonathan Vaughters alluded to earlier, making a leap from the academic environment of the laboratories to the frenzied, uncontrolled world of professional cycling. Application has to usurp the theory. And that could well happen if the price of techniques like brain-imaging drops. In the search for motivation, decision-making and fatigue, just how long will it be before Team Sky riders enter the Death Star through an MRI machine?

# GLOSSARY

**accelerometers** An electro-mechanical device that measures acceleration forces.

**aerobars** Come as one-piece or clip-ons and make the front end of a bike more aerodynamic. The extensions allow the rider to stretch out, creating a lower frontal profile.

**altitude tent** A sealed tent that features reduced oxygen content to simulate a high altitude. Often placed over a rider's bed so they can enjoy physiological adaptations while they sleep.

**anaerobic capacity** The total amount of energy that's obtained from anaerobic sources (without the presence of oxygen) in a single bout of continuous exercise.

**ASO** French company Amaury Sport Organisation organise the Tour de France and are headed up by charismatic director Christian Prudhomme.

**ATP-PC system** Otherwise known as the adenosine triphosphate and phosphocreatine system. This is the body's most immediate energy system through the breakdown of high-energy phosphates. If fully stocked, will provide energy for maximal-intensity, short-duration cycling for 10–15 seconds before fatigue kicks in.

**bidon** A water bottle.

**blood plasma** The pale yellow liquid that contains white blood cells, red blood cells and platelets.

**breakaway** When one rider, or a small group of riders, breaks free from the main peloton. Often instigated by the smaller teams at the Tour to secure TV air time for their sponsors.

**cadence** In cycling terms, the number of revolutions of the crank each minute.

**carbohydrate metabolism** The breakdown of carbohydrates in the mitochondria to produce energy.

**cardiac output** Volume of blood pumped by the heart each minute.

**central nervous system (CNS)** Consists of the brain and spinal cord. When a receptor is stimulated, it sends a signal along the nerve cells (neurons) to the brain.

**chamois pad** The pad either placed or stitched into bike shorts that adds comfort between derrière and saddle.

**compression socks** Tight-fitting socks that purport to increase blood flow from the limbs to the heart, to accelerate the flushing through of oxygen and clear out waste products.

**CompuTrainer** Technologically-advanced indoor cycle trainer.

**cortisol** Often called the 'stress hormone' and produced in the adrenal glands, cortisol influences many of the changes that occur in the body in response to stress including regulating blood-sugar levels.

**cowbells** The soundtrack to the Tour de France!

**crank** Refers to the crank arm, which is the section connected to the pedal.

**directeur sportif** A *directeur sportif* (French for sporting director) directs the team during a race. They follow the team in a car and communicate with the riders, other staff and officials by radio.

**disc wheel** As the name suggests, a wheel that resembles a disc. Usually made of carbon, it features no spokes, the idea being that the lack of spokes increases aerodynamics. Allowed in time trials but banned from mass-start stages due to potential issues with handling in cross winds.

**domestique** A selfless rider who works for the benefit of his team and leader. In French, domestique translates as 'servant'.

**drafting** Where one rider sits directly behind the rider in front. The rider in front acts as a shield from the wind, so reducing air resistance on the rider behind, meaning they enjoy a free ride.

**effector** Any part of the body that produces a response to the receptors. An example would be a muscle contracting to move the legs.

**energy gel** Sachet of carbohydrate – or sometimes carbohydrate plus protein – goo that delivers a burst of energy.

**EPO** Otherwise known as erythro-poietin, it's a hormone that is predominantly produced in the kidneys and is responsible for red blood cell production. A synthetic version was created for patients suffering from anaemia, but was also abused by cyclists to increase their oxygen carrying capacity.

**ergometer** A cycle ergometer is simply an indoor cycle.

**fast-twitch muscles** Muscle fibres that contract quickly to generate high levels of power. On the downside, they fatigue quickly.

**fat metabolism** The break-down of fatty acids in the mitochondria to produce energy.

**fork** The part of the bicycle that holds the front wheel. A steerer tube attaches the fork to the frame and handlebars.

**frontal profile** The profile of the bike and rider as seen from the front, that is, the part that faces the air in front.

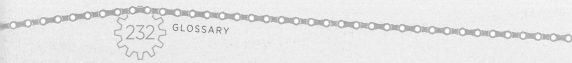

**fructose** A simple sugar that the body can directly use to produce energy.

**functional threshold** The maximum effort a cyclist can maintain for one hour. From this figure, a rider's training zones are set.

**gluconeogenesis** When the body is desperate for energy, it will begin breaking down protein. In essence, the body starts eating itself – muscle – to fuel the session.

**glucose** A simple sugar and one of the primary molecules that provides an energy source for humans. Glycogen is first broken down into glucose before the body breaks it down further for energy.

**glycogen** A multi-branched polysaccharide of glucose that serves as the body's carbohydrate storage system. Glycogen is primarily made and stored in the muscle and liver cells.

**glycogen-depleted sessions** Where you train fasted, so depleting the body's glycogen stores. In turn, the body has to rely on metabolising fat to get through the session.

**green jersey** The jersey awarded to the best sprinter in the Tour. Points are gained for intermediate sprints – sprints within stages – and final position on sprint stages.

**haematocrit** The percentage of red blood cells in blood.

**haemoglobin** Oxygen-carrying protein found in red blood cells.

**headtube** Part of the frame that the fork's steering tube sits in.

**ice vest** A garment similar to a body warmer that features cooling pads and technologies to keep the rider cool before a hot stage.

**internal routing** Where the brake and gear cables run in, rather than on, the frame. Adds to a bike's aerodynamics.

**iron** Iron is used to produce red blood cells.

**isotonic** An isotonic solution contains similar concentrations of salt and sugar as in the human body.

**lactate threshold** Lactate can be recycled in the muscle cells but as exercise intensity increases, levels increase, reaching a tipping point where the lactic acid floods into the bloodstream. This can impair muscle contraction and create that 'burn' feeling. This point is known as the lactate threshold.

**lactic acid** A by-product of the body breaking down carbohydrate for energy without the presence of oxygen.

**maglia rosa** The pink leader's jersey at the Giro d'Italia.

**maltodextrin** A polysaccharide that derives from corn starch.

**MCT** Otherwise known as medum-chain triglycerides, a chain of fatty acids. Some cyclists use MCTs to meet energy demands.

**mitochondria** Organelles found in most cells in which the biochemical processes of respiration and energy production occur. Often known as the powerhouses of the cells.

**muscular endurance** Ability of a muscle or group of muscles to work continuously for a long time without reducing power output through fatigue.

**muscular recruitment** The number of muscles recruited to perform an activity.

**myoglobin** protein in heart and skeletal muscle. When you ride, your muscles use up any available oxygen. Myoglobin has oxygen attached to it, which provides extra oxygen for the muscles to maintain exercise intensity for a longer duration.

**neuromuscular** Relating to nerves and muscles.

**nitric oxide** A key signalling molecule throughout the body. Helps to relax the arteries, so plays a critical role in blood pressure and overall circulation.

**omega-3** Rich form of essential fatty acids found in fish, nuts, flax seed and leafy vegetables. They are a key family of polyunsaturated fats.

**overload** Progressive overload is the gradual increase of stress on the body during exercise, leading to fitness gains.

**oxygen cost** The rate at which the respiratory muscles consume oxygen as they ventilate the lungs.

**palmarès** French for an athlete's list of achievements.

**Paris–Roubaix** Early-April one-day race in Northern France that began in 1896. Also known as the 'Hell of the North' and 'Queen of the Classics' down to its numerous brutal cobbled sections.

**peloton** The main group of riders in a bike race.

**periodisation of nutrition** Where the choice of food matches the intensity of the session or block of training.

**pituitary gland** The major endocrine gland, it's pea-sized and is attached to the base of the brain. It's important in controlling growth and development, and directs the functions of other endocrine glands.

**polyunsaturated fats** A type of good fat found mostly in plant-based foods and oils. Evidence shows that eating foods rich in polyunsaturated fats improves blood cholesterol levels, which can decrease the risk of heart disease.

**power meter** A training tool that measures a cyclist's power output. Measurement commonly takes place in the bottom bracket, crank arm or pedal.

**protein synthesis** The process whereby cells generate new proteins. An important component of muscle repair after exercise.

**puncheur** A rider who specialises in courses that feature short, sharp hills, like those encountered in races like Liège–Bastogne–Liège.

**quadriceps** A group of four muscles located in the front of the thigh. The Latin translation of quadriceps is 'four-headed', as the group contains four separate muscles: vastus lateralis, vastus medialis, vastus intermedius and rectus femoris.

**receptors** A group of specialised cells that detect changes in their environment, which are called 'stimuli', and turn them into electrical impulses.

**red blood cells** Also called erythrocytes, they are round with a flattish, indented centre like a doughnut without a hole. Their principal role is to deliver oxygen around the body and carry carbon dioxide to the lungs.

**reticulocyte** An immature red blood cell. Reticulocytes commonly compose about 1 per cent of the red blood cells in the human body.

**rouleur** An all-rounder who performs well on all types of course, though often works as a domestique for his team leader.

**saddle sore** A skin ailment often of the buttocks, deriving from excessive friction between buttocks and saddle.

**seat tube** The frame tube running from the bottom bracket up to either the seatpost or, if the frame features a seat tube and post in one, the saddle.

**slow-twitch muscles** Muscle fibres that contract slowly but can keep going for a long time.

**stem** The bike component that attaches the handlebars to the frame.

**taper** Where you reduce the volume of cycling in the lead-up to a goal race. The aim? To be at your optimum fitness.

**testosterone** A steroid that's produced in the testes (men), ovaries (women) and adrenal glands (both). In cycling terms, testosterone is important to red blood cell production and muscle strength.

**thermal regulation** Otherwise known as temperature regulation, this refers to the body's core temperature, which usually measures 37°C. Not overheating during exercise is one of the body's primary aims, especially when cycling in the heat.

**tidal volume** The amount of air breathed in or out of the lungs in one breath.

**time trial** Known as the purest form of road cycling as it's rider against the clock.

**Tour of Lombardy** The final one-day classic of the season takes place in early October in Italy, hence its nickname 'Race of the Falling Leaves'.

**tri-spokes** A wheel that comprises just three carbon spokes, though they are much wider than traditional spokes. The idea is that fewer spokes equals less choppy air equals less drag … equals more speed.

**tryptophan** An amino acid that your body must get from its diet. The body uses tryptophan to help make niacin and serotonin. Serotonin is thought to be responsible for healthy sleep and a stable mood. Milk is a good source of tryptophan.

**UCI** The Union Cycliste Internationale is the international governing body of cycling. Their headquarters are in Aigle, Switzerland.

**VO$_2$ max** A measure of the maximum volume of oxygen that an athlete can use each minute. It is measured in millilitres per kilogram of body weight.

**vortices** As a cyclist moves through the air, he produces a turbulent wake behind him. These are vortices, which create a low-pressure area behind the cyclist and an area of wind that moves along with the cyclist. If you're behind this cyclist, you can draft in this low pressure and conserve energy at no cost to speed.

**WADA** Otherwise known as the World Anti-Doping Agency. The body was set up in 1999 by a collective initiative led by the International Olympic Committee. WADA is responsible for the World Anti-Doping Code, which has been adopted by more than 600 sports organisations, and determines which performance enhancers might be deemed legal or illegal.

**watts** The standard measurement of power.

**wheel rim** The outer edge of the wheel that holds the tyre and spokes. Rim depth can influence how much drag is created. A shallower rim is less aerodynamic than a deep rim, though does create a lighter wheel. Time trials use deep rims; mountain stages tend to attract shallower versions.

**wind-chill** Bike speed creates the same environmental effect as wind speed, and the greater the wind speed, the colder it is. If it's a relatively balmy 8°C and you're cycling at 25km/h, it'll feel like a whisker over 4°C. Crank up to 40km/h and it'll feel like 3°C. That's bearable. But if the temperature drops to 2°C at both speeds, then wind-chill makes it feel nearer −3°C and −5°C, respectively.

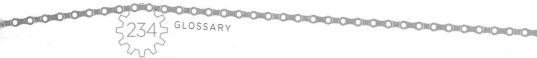

# INDEX

*Page numbers with 'g' are terms also found in the glossary.*

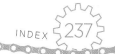

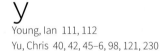

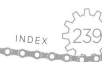

# PICTURE CREDITS

All photographs © Getty Images with the following exceptions:

Page 33 © Grant Pritchard
Pages 34,35 © BrakeThrough Media
Page 30 © Carson Blume
Page 37 © Cervelo
Pages 40,42,89 © Trek Factory Racing
Pages 52,136,195,218 © Wouter Roosenboom
Page 99 © Specialized
Pages 161,172,186-187,192,206 © Graham Watson
Page 221 © BMC Racing Team

## Acknowledgements

○ There are many people to thank for making my job writing *The Science of The Tour de France* that bit easier and much more interesting. Firstly, it's hard to ignore ASO. They organise the Tour de France, without which this book would of course never been written!

Thank you to all the sports scientists, nutritionists, chefs, physiologists, DSes, riders, press contacts and many more who offered their time and knowledge. In particular, sincere gratitude to Daniel Healey, David Bailey, David Martin and Michael Rogers, who put up with my endless questions on countless occasions.

Bloomsbury for showing such enthusiasm and encouragement throughout. Special mentions to Charlotte for her searing honesty, commitment and comments; Sarah for politely haranguing and driving the project forward when my email responses were slower than slow; and the copyeditor, proofreader and art crew who beautified many of my ramblings.

To all the magazine editors I've continued to contribute to with while writing this book, especially *Cyclist*'s Pete Muir, who politely accepted my late filings of work. Hopefully the content eclipsed the lateness!

The family Witts-Morse for always being rather brilliant, especially my son Harry, whose insistence on playing football kept me sane (not to mention his great *The Science of The Tour de France* cover mock-ups), and my daughter Mia, whose knowledge of science will take her further than she feels possible. Mother and father for being the best parents a Devon lad could wish for – and, of course, for buying my blue pearlescent Peugeot bicycle when I was young. And my sister for providing timely boosts when the finish line seemed further away than the peak of Alpe d'Huez.

Finally, my wife Tara for tolerating missed weekends, evenings and early mornings while I wrote, fretted and was generally a bit of a pain. Your support, confidence and love for me made this happen. You are the best.